ORGANIC BEAUTY RECIPES
By Eve

THE COMPLETE GUIDE TO DIY NATURAL BEAUTY

Eve Cabanel
www.organic-beauty-recipes.com

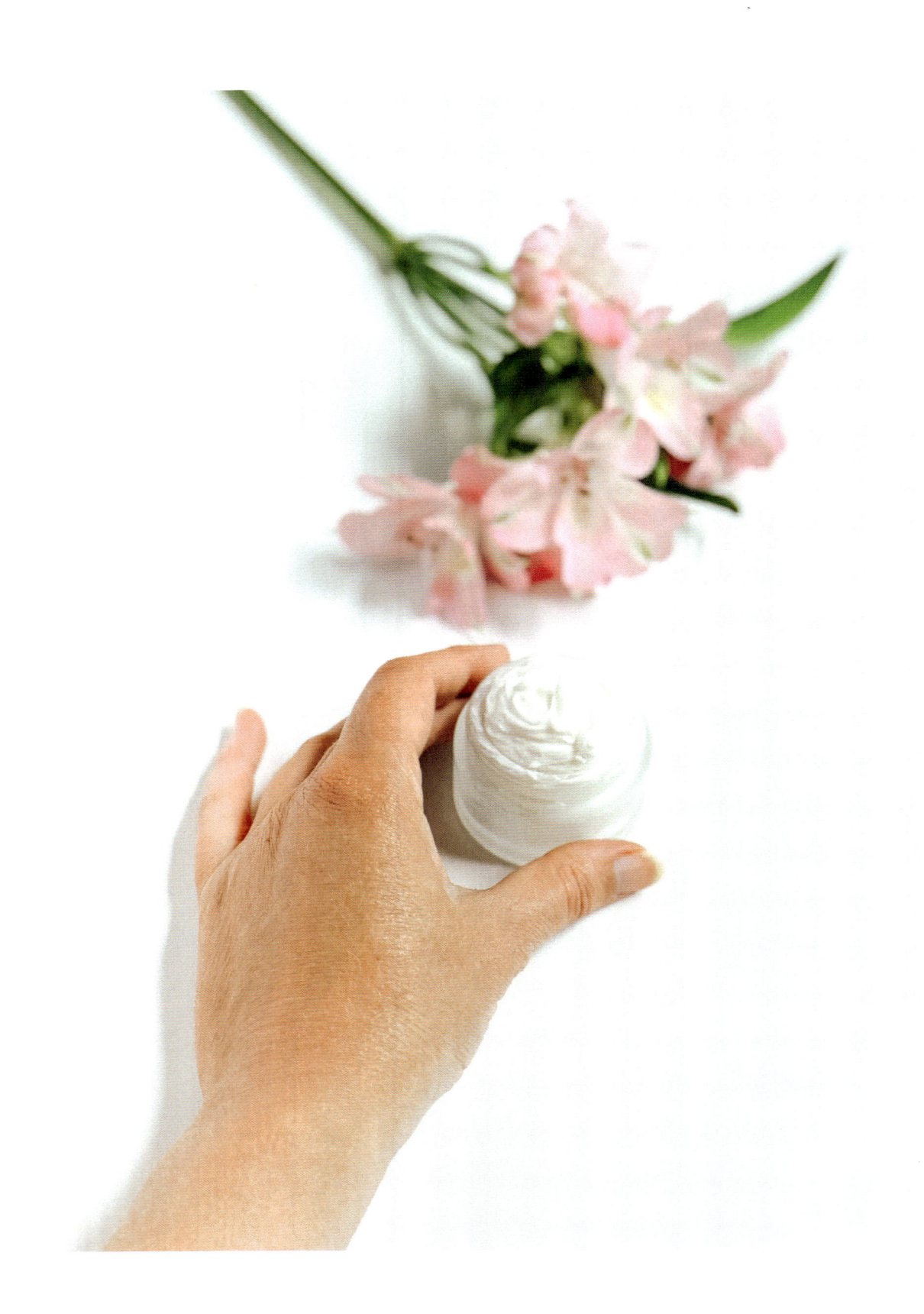

PRAISES

"Natural is best ... Organic even better! All of the organic beauty recipes are easy to follow and use ingredients that are readily available. What we put in our bodies is important but equally important is what we put on our bodies. Organic-beauty-recipes.com is a great website, informative and one of the first places I visit when I'm looking for DIY beauty recipes. Inspirational!"

Michelle Norris
– Harvest, USA

"Eve's recipes have transformed my skincare and my skin! After two decades of struggling with skin that was both eczema-prone and acne-prone, my skin is now healing and glowing! I have stopped purchasing products sold in stores and now make my own simple, healthy, skin-friendly beauty products. I also love that this has a huge environmental impact, with less packaging, so much less waste, and no chemicals or synthetic ingredients. My skin is glowing, I'm saving money, and I'm respecting the Earth. I'm so happy I found Eve's beauty recipes!"

Teresa McWilliam
- Powell River, CANADA

"I love Eve's organic recipes, the instructions are always easy to follow and the results are really impressive."

Amalia Rosoiu. Cirencester, GREAT BRITAIN

"Eve's recipes are not only easy to make and environmentally conscious, they really smell and feel divine and best of all, they work!!"

Brandie Alexander
– Bridgetown, AUSTRALIA

"When you embark to do your own self care products you can find a lot of options and recipes on Internet, but finding ones that REALLY WORK, which gives you substitutions for things you may not have or find, that are created by someone who knows the effects they will produce and what is more suitable for each skin type, that's really difficult. Not with Eve, though. I have had great success with all her recipes, they turn out perfect (which is also cost saving, as you don't have to throw away any ruined project), so I trust her completely. If you are into DIY, don't hesitate to get this book, you won't regret it!!!"

Mary Herald
- Buenos Aires, ARGENTINA

"Eve's beautiful enriching ingredients all from natural sources are wonderfully nourishing on the skin. You know that you're putting goodness on your body with Eve's recipes. And they're very easy to follow and make. My skin is glowing and youthful looking now. I highly recommend Eve's no harmful chemicals, just pure natural ingredients and fabulous recipes to make your own products!"

Suzi Woodfield
– Christchurch, NEW ZEALAND

Written and edited by Eve Cabanel, 1978
@ Copyrights by Eve Cabanel.
All rights reserved. This book or any portion thereof may not be reproduced or used in any manner whatsoever without the express written permission of the author except for the use of brief quotations in a book review.
All images photography are copyrighted by Eve Cabanel except the following:
Image page 18 @ Anna - Adobe Stock Licence
Image page 22 @ Pixel-Shot - Adobe Stock Licence
Image page 24 @ luisapuccini - Adobe Stock Licence
Image page 28 @ New Africa - Adobe Stock Licence
Image page 30 @ nikilitov - Adobe Stock Licence
Image page 36 @ pamela_d_mcadams - Adobe Stock Licence
Image page 66 @ floraldeco - Adobe Stock Licence
Image page 68 @ tstock - Adobe Stock Licence
Image page 84 @ Flaffy - Adobe Stock Licence
Image page 122 @ Jiri Hera - Adobe Stock Licence

Publisher's Cataloging-in-Publication data
Eve Cabanel
Title: Organic Beauty Recipes By Eve – The complete guide to DIY natural beauty
www.organic-beauty-recipes.com

ISBN: 9798645375072
Imprint: Independently published by Amazon
1. Beauty, Crafts.
2. Herbal cosmetics.

First Edition, September 2020

THIS BOOK IS DEDICATED TO

My better half Paul
Who supported me during all those years...
May we continue to grow together,
May our love expand to the universe and back!

You my reader
May you find the strength to follow a healthy natural beauty routine & lifestyle,
Closer to nature and in touch with your mind, body and soul...
May you be inspired and create amazing DIY beauty recipes!

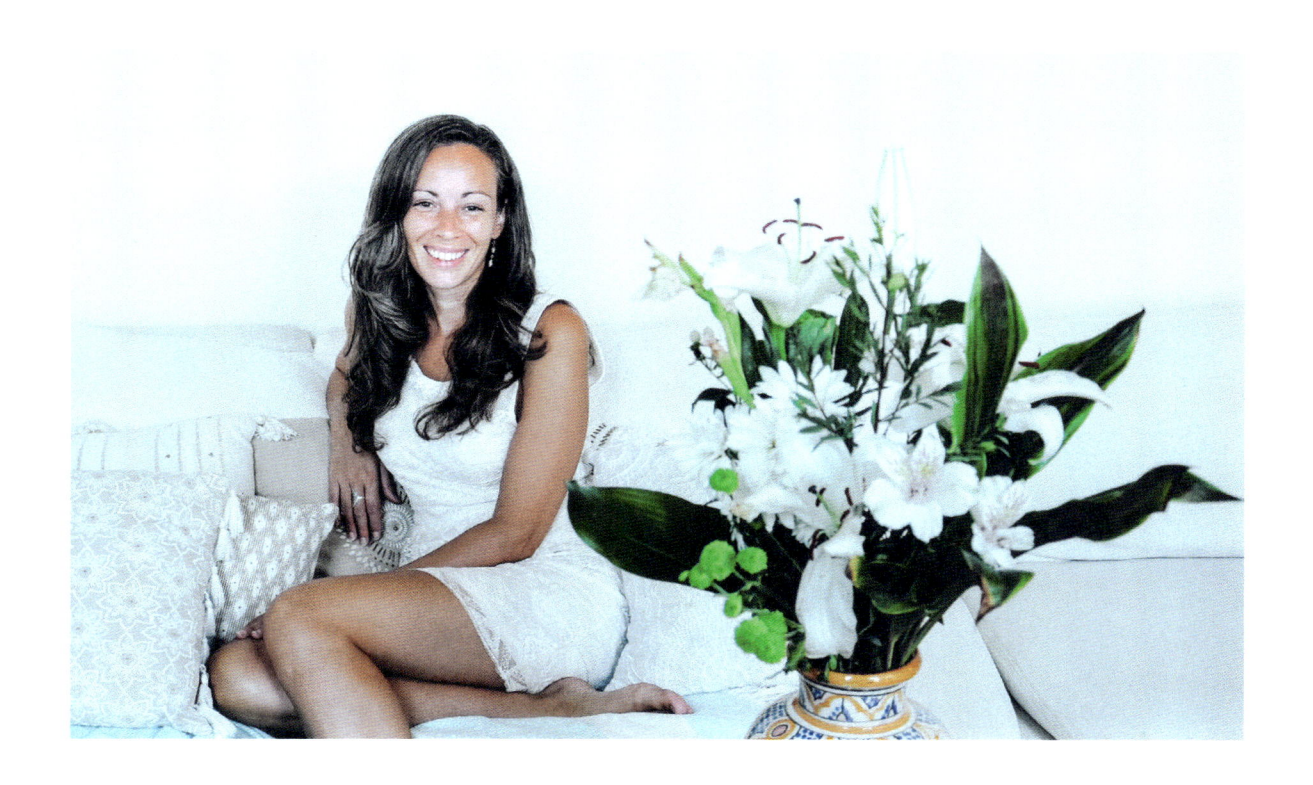

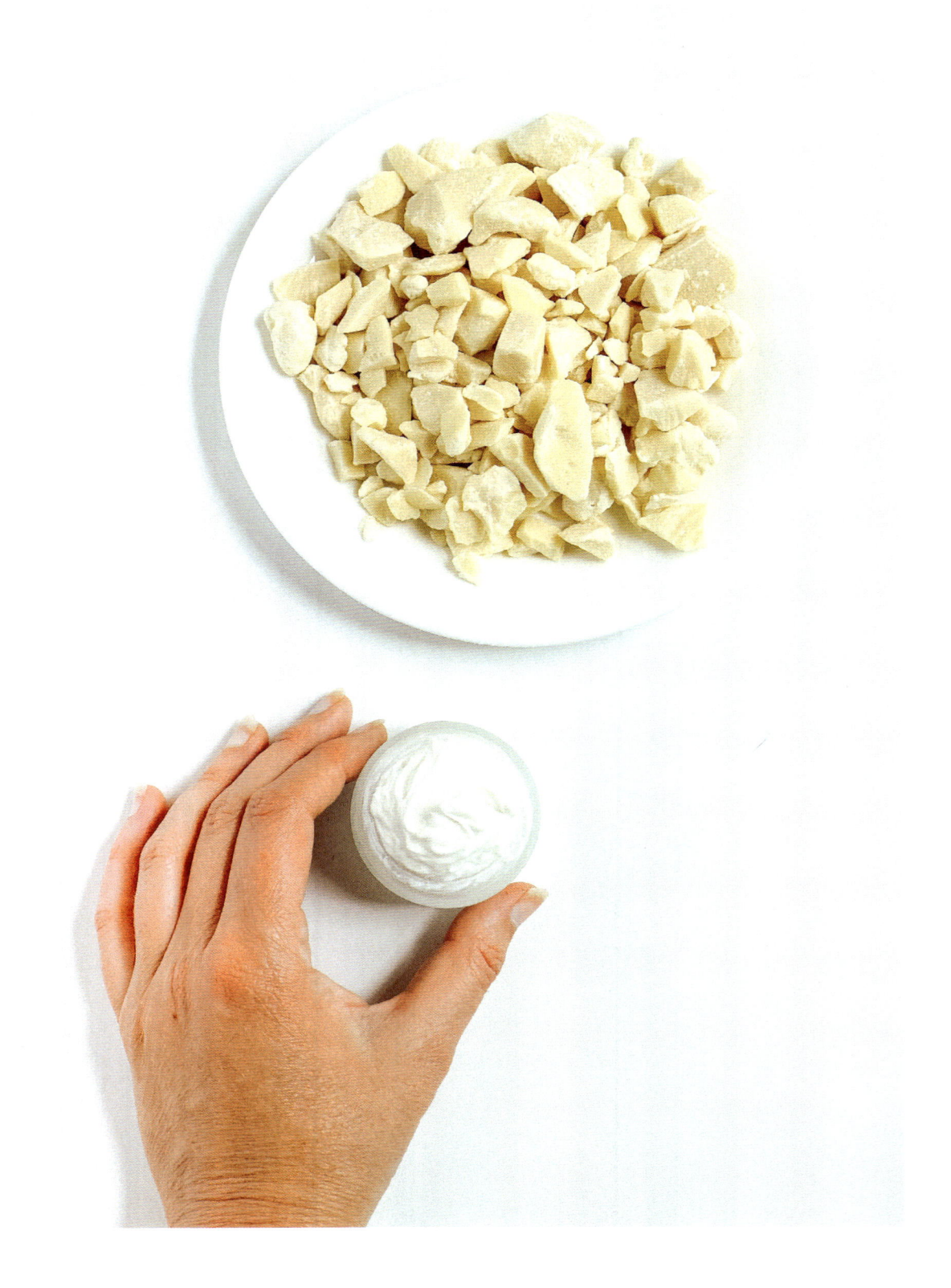

CONTENTS

INTRO — 13
My Mission & Vision — 13
My promise to you — 13
My journey to natural beauty — 13
A wake-up call — 16
Is buying natural beauty products the solution? — 16
Why use organic ingredients? — 17
Join Our growing Organic Beauty Recipes Community — 17

Chapter 1 – THE ESSENTIALS — 21

CARRIER OILS — 21
Jojoba oil — 21
Sunflower oil — 21
Rosehip oil — 22
Sacha Inchi Oil — 22
Kukui Nut oil — 22
Coconut oil — 22
Camellia seed oil — 23

BUTTERS — 25
Shea butter — 25
Cocoa butter — 25
Mango butter — 25
Ucuuba butter — 25
Kokum butter — 25

HYDROSOLS AND FLOWER WATER — 27
Orange blossom hydrosol — 27
Rosewater or rose hydrosol — 27
Chamomile hydrosol — 27

ALOE VERA — 29
How to prepare aloe vera gel from fresh leaves — 29
Aloe vera healing cleanser and after sun soother — 31

ESSENTIAL OILS — 33
- Lavender essential oil — 33
- Roman Chamomile essential oil — 33
- Frankincense essential oil — 33
- Peppermint essential oil — 33
- Rose Geranium essential oil — 33

NATURAL EMULSIFIERS — 35
- What is an emulsion? — 35
- Beeswax — 35
- Rice Bran Wax — 35
- Liquid Lecithin — 37
- Naturally-derived emulsifier — 37

NATURAL PRESERVATIVES — 39
- When to use Natural Preservatives in your homemade beauty products? — 39
- Top 3 Natural preservatives in DIY Beauty — 41
- Rosemary oil extract — 41
- Grapefruit seed extract — 41
- Essential oils — 41
- Why I don't use chemical preservatives — 41
- How to make sure your homemade beauty products don't spoil? — 42
- The controversy over DIY and preservatives — 42

EQUIPMENT TO GET STARTED — 45
- My top 5 basic Equipment for DIY Beauty Products — 45

CONTAINERS — 49
- Body butter and creams — 49
- Containers for Essential Oil blends or perfumes — 49
- Containers for serums — 51
- Containers for homemade Lip balms — 51
- Substitutions in DIY beauty products — 52
- 1. The speed of a carrier oil absorption in the skin — 52
- 2. The texture of the oil or butter — 53
- 3. The Melting point — 54

Chapter 2 – DIY BODY CARE PRODUCTS					57

    BODY BUTTER RECIPES						59
    SHEA BODY BUTTER RECIPE WITH ONLY 2 INGREDIENTS		59
    WHIPPED SHEA BODY BUTTER					61
    MANGO BODY BUTTER						63
    COCOA BODY BUTTER RECIPE					65
    COCONUT BODY BUTTER						67

    BODY CREAM RECIPES						69
    GALEN COLD CREAM						69
    HOMEMADE BODY CREAM TUTORIAL					71
    HAND LOTION FOR DRY HANDS (PUMPABLE!)				75

    MASSAGE BAR RECIPES						77
    HOW TO MAKE LOTION BARS WITOUT BEESWAX			77
    DIY COFFEE MASSAGE BAR AGAINST CELLULITE			79
    HOMEMADE LOTION BAR FOR DRY SKIN				81
    DIY MASSAGE BAR FOR SORE MUSLES				83

    BODY SCRUB RECIPES						85
    COCONUT AND PINEAPLE BODY SCRUB				85
    COFFEE BODY SCRUB						87
    HYMALAYAN SEA SALT FOOD SCRUB & SOAK				89

    DEODORANT							91
    HOMEMADE DEODORANT WITHOUT BAKING SODA			91

    SUNCREENS							93
    HOMEMADE SUNSCREEN WITHOUT TITANIUM DIOXIDE			93

    TEETH AND GUM NATURAL CARE					95
    DIY PEPPERMINT TOOTHPASTE					95

Chapter 3 – DIY FACE CARE PRODUCTS					97

    FACE CREAM RECIPES						99
    ROSE FACE CREAM						99
    FACE MOISTURIZER WITH ROYAL JELLY				101
    FACE CREAM WITH SACHA INCHI OIL FOR MATURE SKIN		105

DIY MAKE UP REMOVER CREAM	107
ANTI AGING FACE CREAM WITHOUT BEESWAX	109
FACE SERUMS	111
OIL CLEANSING METHOD FOR ACNE	111
What is the OCM Method?	111
Benefits of the Oil Cleansing Method for Acne	111
HOMEMADE FACE SERUM FOR OILY SKIN	113
HOMEMADE FACE SERUM FOR DRY SKIN	115
DIY FACE SERUM RECIPE ANTI WRINKLES	117
FACE SCRUBS	119
FACE SCRUB WITH APRICOT KERNEL POWDER	119
MATCHA SUGAR SCRUB	121
ADZUKI BEAN FACE SCRUB	123
COFFEE FACE SCRUB RECIPE	125
DIY FACE MASKS	127
DIY CHARCOAL MASK	127
CLAY MASK RECIPE FOR ACNE	129
AYURVEDIC FACE MASK	131
DIY LIP CARE PRODUCTS	132
LIP BALM RECIPES	133
COCONUT OIL LIP BALM	133
HONEY LIP BALM	135
VEGAN LIP BALM WITHOUT BEESWAX	137
TINTED LIP BALM WITH COCONUT OIL AND SOYWAX	139
HOMEMADE PEPPERMINT LIP BALM	143
LIP GLOSS RECIPES	145
HOW TO MAKE PINK LIP GLOSS WITH BEETROOT	145
HONEY LIP GLOSS	147
Tutorial DIY honey lip gloss	149
LIPSTICK RECIPES	151
HOW TO MAKE LIPSTICK LIKE A PRO	151
Tutorial - How to use the lipstick silicon mold	153
DIY MATTE LIPSTICK WITHOUT BEESWAX	155
INDEX	157

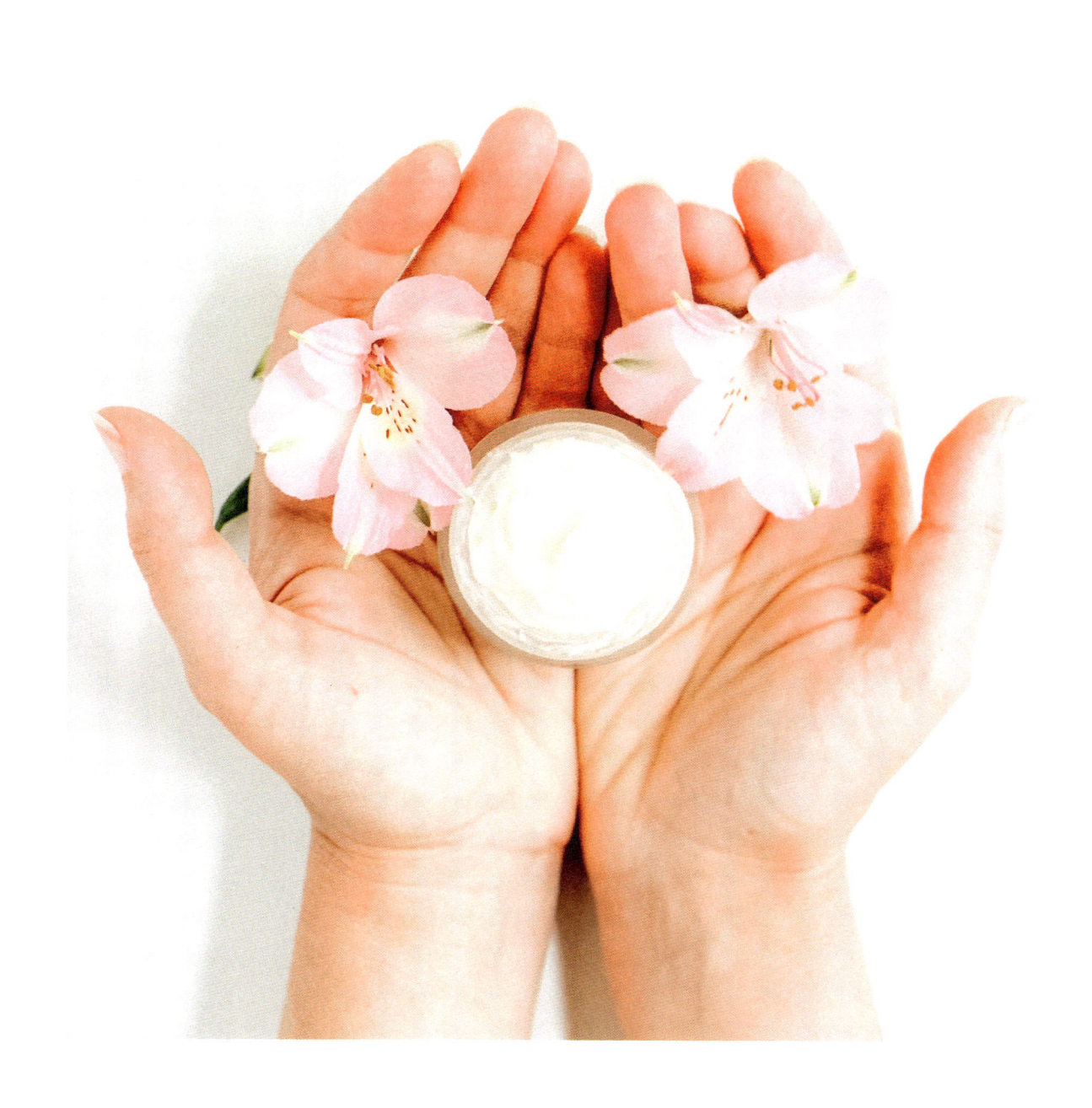

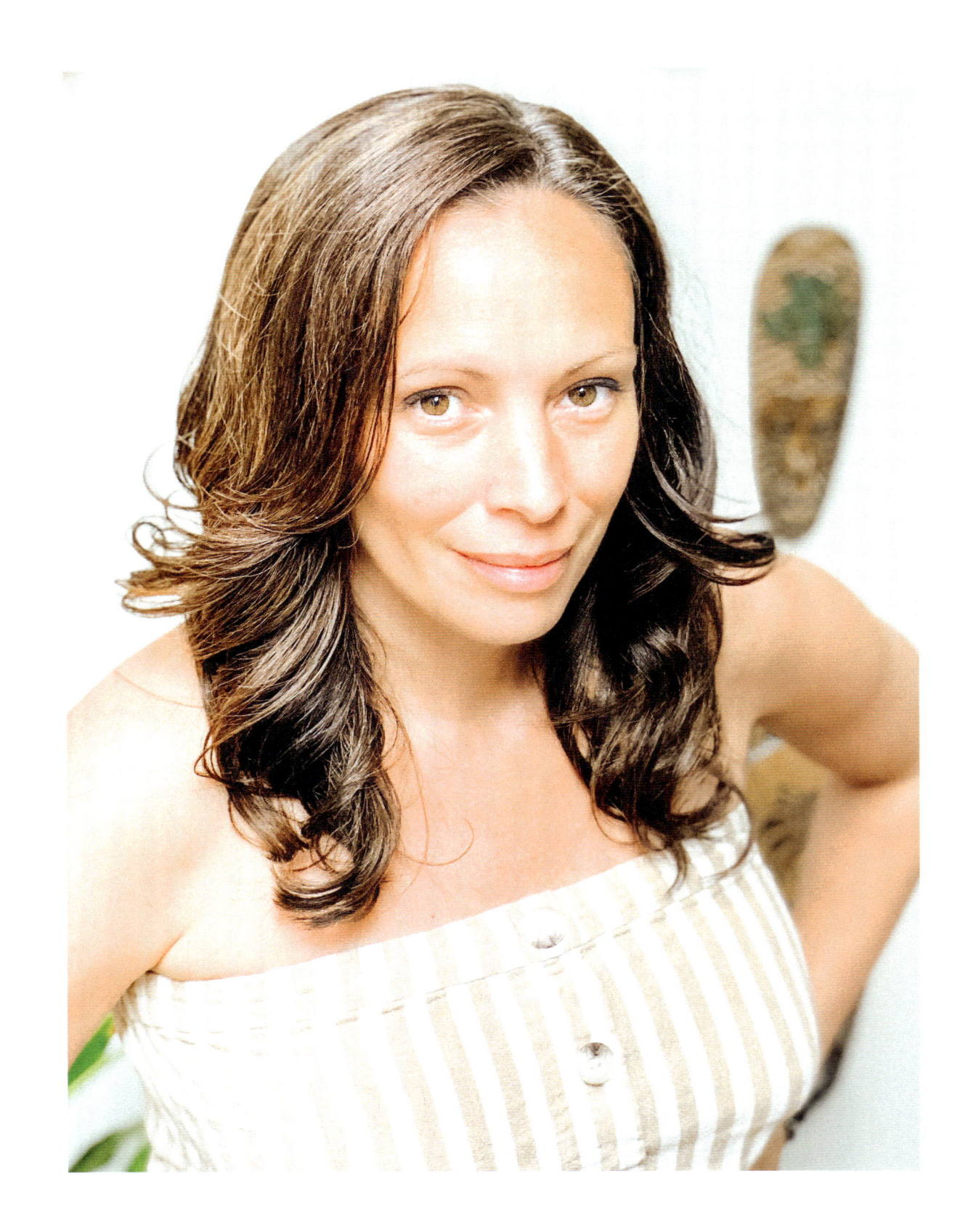

INTRO

I'm Eve, homemade DIY organic skincare recipe creator. So glad you have decided to take steps towards DIY natural beauty!

Hard to believe but this book is 10 years in the making and contains my most popular organic beauty recipes. I carefully craft and test all the recipes you will find in this book!

I created my blog http://www.organic-beauty-recipes.com in 2010 when I started researching the ingredients in my daily commercial beauty products and was shocked to learn about the harmful effects on my health.

My Mission
I've embarked on a journey to empower women on how they can make their own organic beauty recipes at home and make the switch towards a healthier lifestyle.

My Promise to You
I will be revealing some fabulous homemade organic beauty products recipes that have been tried and tested at home (on humans!).

Homemade face & body creams, body butters, lip balms, cleansers, natural perfumes & makeup won't be a secret to you anymore. And I will do my best to make them easy and fun... oh and yes, it will save you a TON of money in the process.

Why Go Organic & Homemade?
- **ORGANIC** = *Grown or made without the use of chemicals like pesticides, insecticides or fungicides*
- **BEAUTY** = *Attractive, healthy, I mean... beauty inside out!*
- **RECIPES** = *Easy and homemade right in my kitchen*

By whipping up your own natural beauty products, you are making a statement that you do not want to support dangerous commercial beauty products filled with chemicals that are linked to cancer, hormone disruptions, and other health problems...

My favorite expression: *"Be the change you want to see in the world!"* Every little action counts!

My journey to natural beauty
In 2009, I lost my beloved grandmother "Mamie" to cancer. It was the first time I lost someone really close to me that I deeply felt connected with. She was this strong-minded yet calm, cheerful woman that exulted kindness.

She taught me how to ride a bike and was the one who always fired up my imagination as a child by telling me made up stories, one including a tale with an adventurous flea with tennis shoes...!

14   ORGANIC BEAUTY RECIPES BY EVE

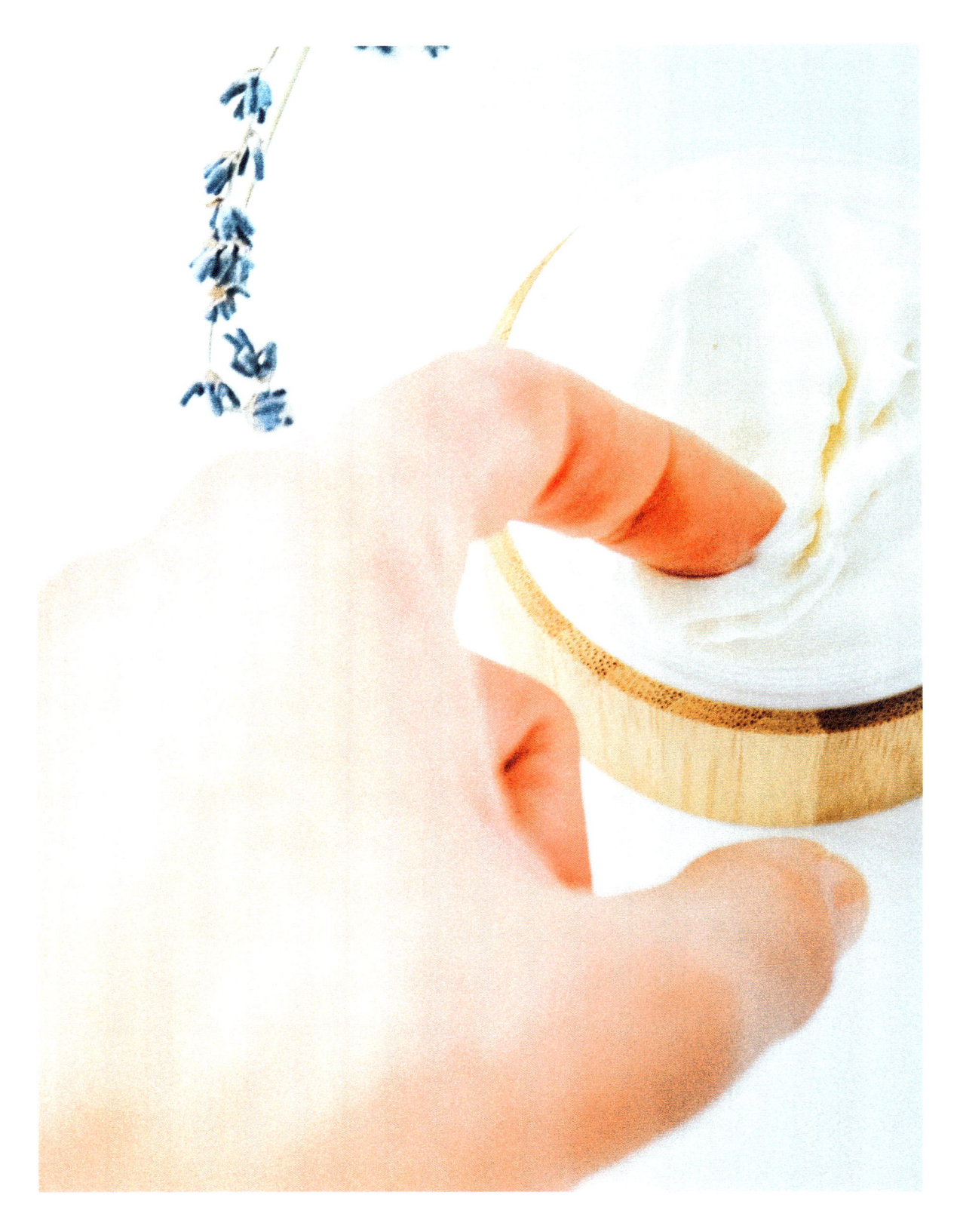

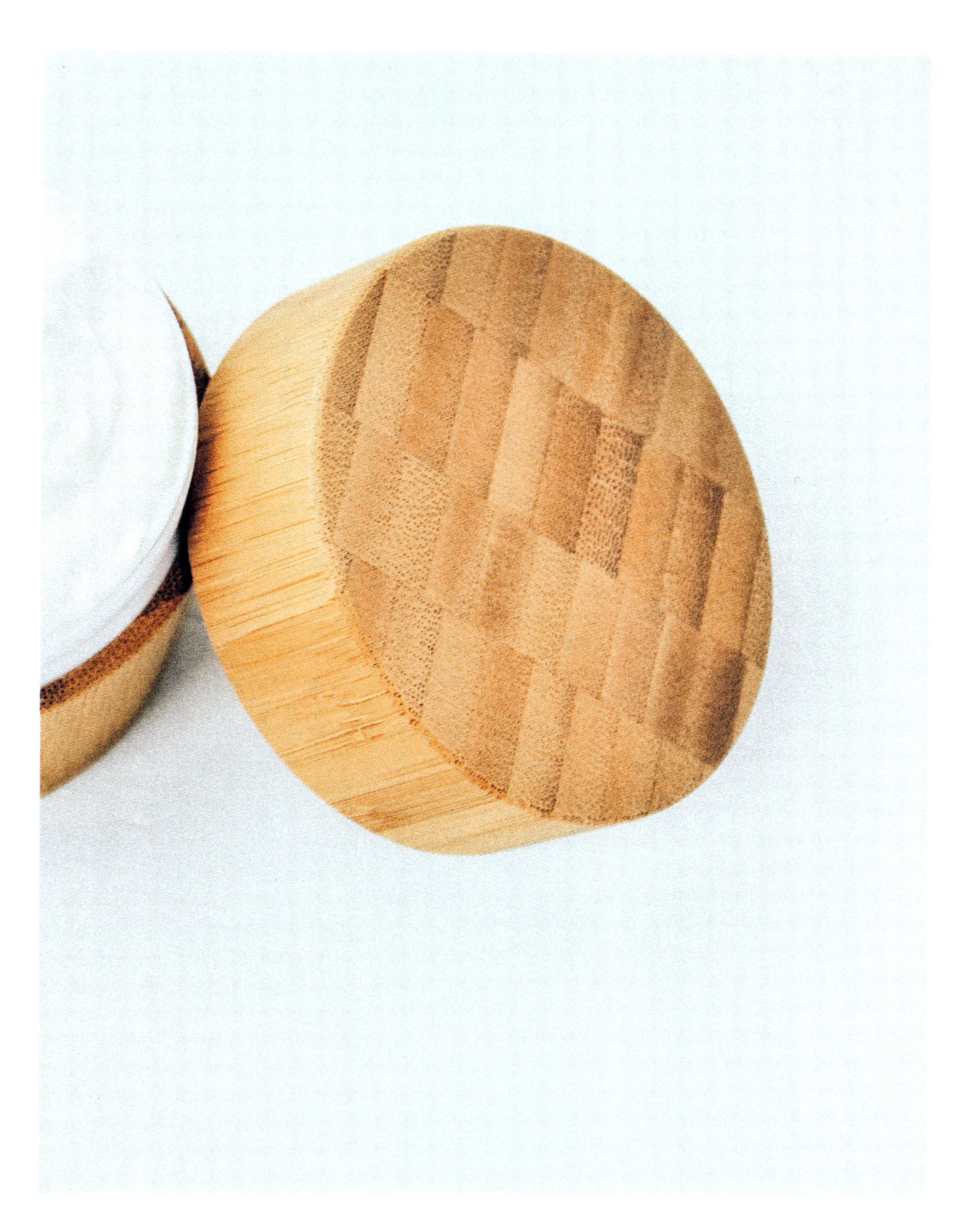

A wake-up call

Her loss was a wake-up call for me. I researched the ingredients in my daily commercial beauty products and was baffled that I could not understand their meaning. While looking at each ingredient on the website and database of Skin Deep, I was shocked to learn about the harmful effects these chemicals have on our health, as well as the lack of studies and research available on some ingredients.

I had used a popular commercial brand of deodorant and soap for years and now realized how dangerous the ingredients were for my health, especially since I was using them daily. For many years, I battled with acne and also developed intolerance to commercial synthetic perfumes.

Example of dangerous ingredients
- Methyl, ethyl, propyl, benzyl and butyl parabens - **hormone disrupter, linked to breast cancer**
- Aluminum chloralhydrate, aluminum zirconium tetrachlorohydrex gly - **linked to breast cancer**
- Propylene Glycol - **delayed allergic reactions, possible kidney, and liver damage**
- BHT - **irritation, developmental/reproductive toxicity, linked to cancer**
- Fragrance (pretty much in ALL commercial beauty products unless fragrance-free!) – **skin irritation, harmful to the environment, allergies and organ system toxicity**

Why would our society allow commercial companies to put a product in the market that is dangerous or without any long term studies on our health?

The answer is simple: **short term profit and gain vs long term health.**

Is buying natural beauty products the solution?

I then started buying organic certified products but found them to be too costly and was convinced that there should be an easier and simpler solution. Unfortunately, a lot of the certified organic beauty products or so called natural products still use fragrances and chemical preservatives so they can stay on the shelves for years. And please don't get me started on the misleading marketing labels or certifications that claim to be "natural". This is when I finally decided to make the switch and started crafting organic beauty products at home.

And to be honest, nothing is more fulfilling than having total control and using high-quality organic and fair trade ingredients while making your own customized DIY beauty skincare product!

Why use organic ingredients?

While organic ingredients might end up costing you a little more, their benefits far outweigh the cost.

- Organic farmed ingredients don't have a negative impact on the environment (no use of pesticides, fungicides, insecticides).
- Your skin will thank you for using organic ingredients. Being the largest organ in the body, your skin absorbs everything that you apply right into your bloodstream. You don't want absorbing the nasty chemicals found in conventional and non-certified organic ingredients.
- Using organic materials means that you don't run the risk of using GMOs.
- Organic means higher quality. And your skin and your health deserve nothing less than that.

Join Our growing Organic Beauty Recipes Community

Our community is growing, and hundreds of thousands like you are looking for a natural alternative to commercial beauty products! And I know there are more of us going through the same journey I did years ago and wanting to make a change in lifestyle. I love to be part of this awakening!

Get started by signing up to my weekly newsletter on my blog **www.organic-beauty-recipes.com** and join us on Facebook, Instagram, Pinterest for more inspiration.

Don't hesitate to say hi on the above social media channels and if you have any questions; I will do my best to get back to you!

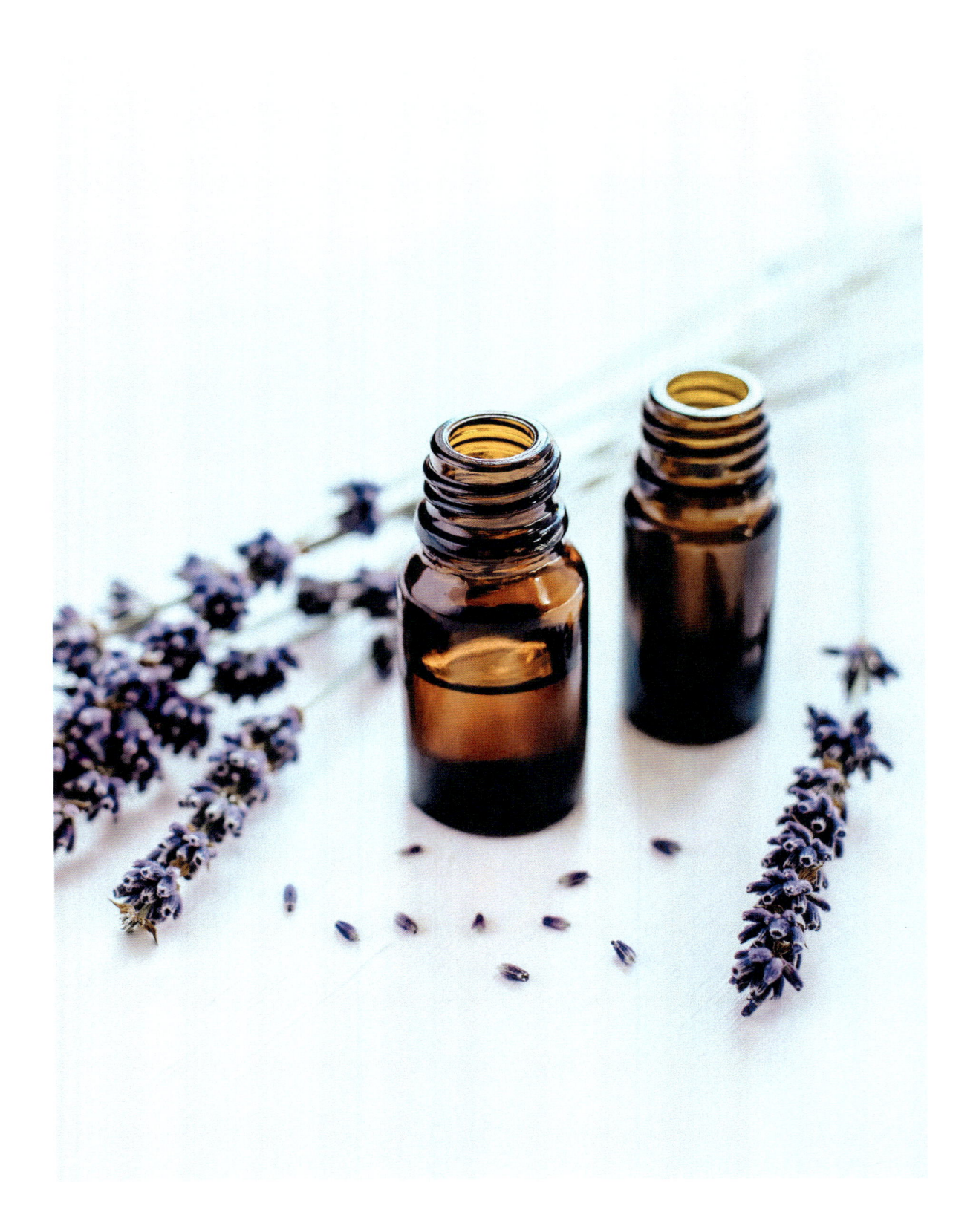

1 THE ESSENTIALS

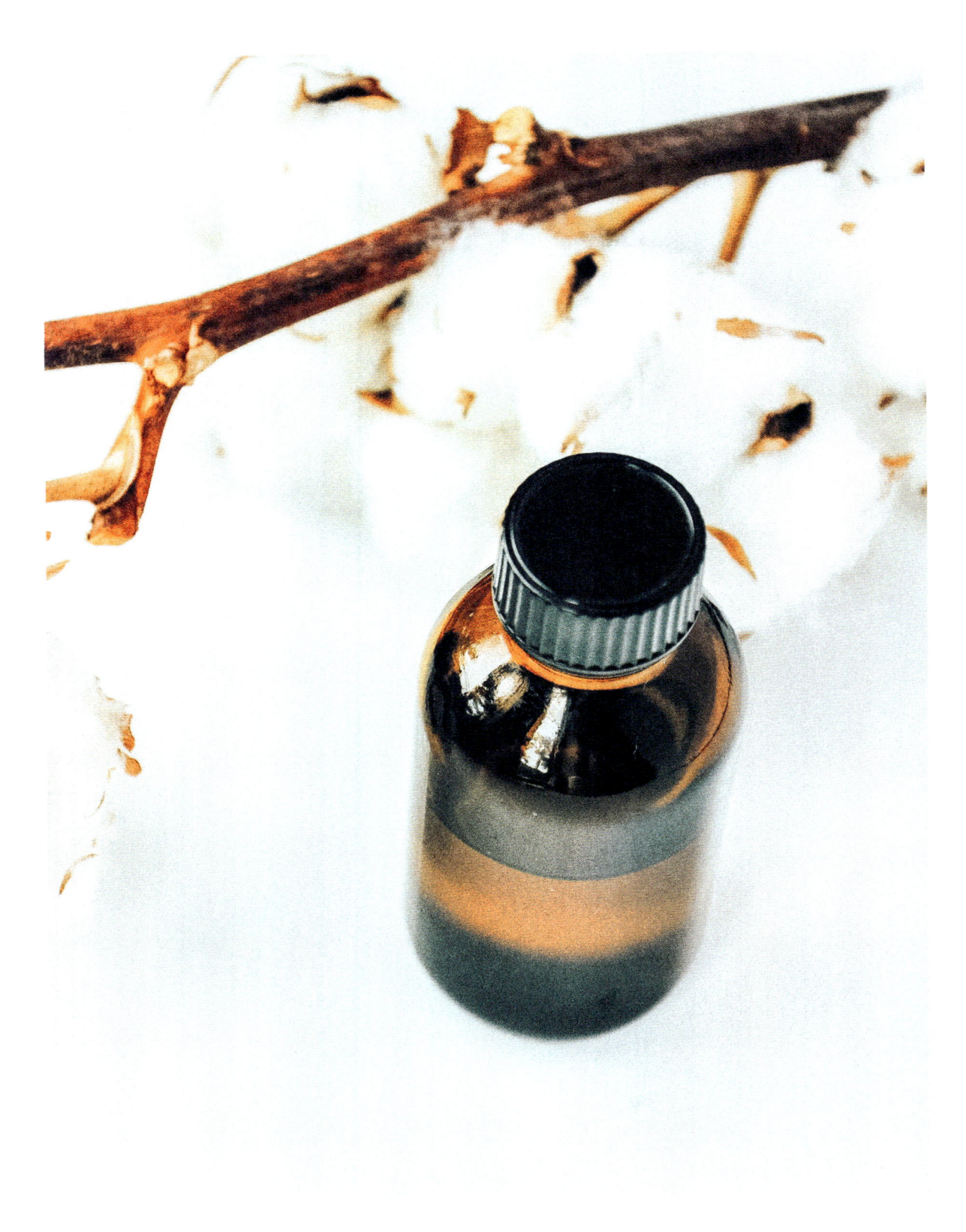

CARRIER OILS

THE ESSENTIALS

Carrier oils are an important part of your DIY beauty arsenal. These versatile oils help to deliver the nutrient-packed benefits of essential oils while providing a mega-dose of hydration and nourishment.

My favorite oils to use in DIY recipes are organic and nutrient-rich. They include jojoba oil, sunflower oil, rosehip oil, coconut oil, avocado oil, argan oil, and camellia seed oil.

You can choose your carrier oil based on a number of factors like absorption rate, viscosity, and nutrient composition. There are fast-absorbing, medium-absorbing and slow-absorbing oils. Each type has its own benefits and you can select which ones you want to use in your recipes depending on your needs and skin type.

How to choose organic carrier oils

There are a number of things to consider when choosing organic carrier oils.

First, look for quality and purity above anything else. Your carrier oil should contain only one ingredient – the oil itself!

Some may contain Vitamin E, but for the most part, you only want to see only one ingredient. Be especially wary of oils that prominently display one ingredient, like argan oil, on the front of the container, but contain a number of chemicals in the ingredients list.

Choose oils that are organic to eliminate contamination by other toxins, such as those in pesticides that may be used on non-organic plants. Many oils are also harvested from plants in developing countries, so look for Fair Trade labels to ensure that the farmers who harvest the crops are compensated fairly.

When you buy organic carrier oils, ensure they are certified with either the organic USDA seal or the ECOCERT seal, this guarantee a thorough process and verification that the oil is actually organic.

You also want to make sure that whichever oil you choose is not extremely expensive, unless you use it sparingly on your face.

Jojoba oil

jojoba oil is oil pressed from the seed of the jojoba plant, which is a shrub found in Mexico and the southwest of the United States. It's high in antioxidants A and E, which help to nourish and moisturize the skin. It is also lightweight and is easily absorbed and is my favorite oil to use on my face daily.

Sunflower oil

sunflower oil is cost efficient, practically unscented and has moisturizing and skin conditioning properties. It is also high in vitamin E which helps prevent sun damage and skin irritation. It's great to use on your body in a body butter recipe.

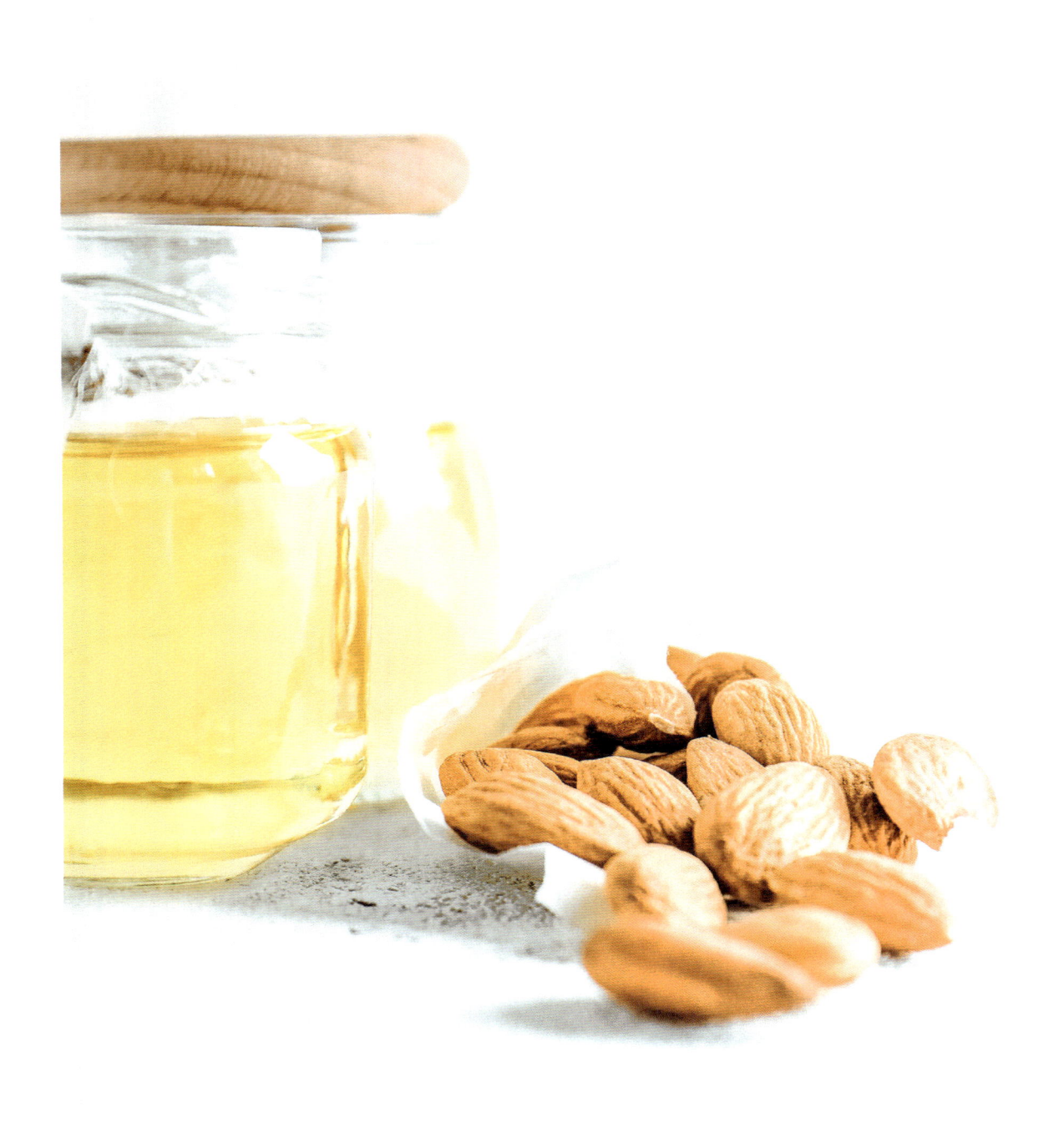

Rosehip oil

Rosehip oil comes from the seeds of rosehip fruit from Chile.

It has a smooth and thin texture and is not greasy. The best quality rosehip oil has an orange and almost red color. It will not color your skin but can help give you a healthy tanned glow naturally.

Rosehip oil is filled with vitamins, antioxidants and fatty acids that hydrate the skin, repair damage from free radicals, reduce skin discoloration.

Keep in mind that not all rosehip oils are created equal. To ensure that you are using the highest quality, you should look for two things in the label—cold-pressed and certified organic. Cold pressed is the best extraction method because it ensures the maximum vitamin content and potency of the oil.

It is great to reduce skin redness and uneven skin tone as well. It's also excellent for sun damaged skins and on your face to smooth out wrinkles.

The price of a 30 ml bottle ranges from $15 to $45 and you can buy it online.

Sacha Inchi Oil

Sacha inchi oil is a superfood that is high in protein, fatty acids, and antioxidants. It mostly contains the antioxidants Vitamin C and Vitamin E, which help to fight free radical damage and counteract aging, making this oil ideal for mature skin. It also has a high fatty acid content of 93% – and most of these fatty acids are in the form of linoleic acid. Linoleic acid is especially beneficial for uneven skin tone and those who are prone to clogged pores.

Sacha inchi oil has a distinctive green and moss-like smell which is why I like to use essential oils to cover the smell. It goes on smooth and absorbs into the skin quickly, creating a protective moisture-locking barrier.

Kukui Nut oil

Kukui nut oil is also one of my favorite oil; I often use it pure and undiluted in the morning on my face. For hundreds of years, Hawaiians have used kukui nut oil for its moisturising and healing properties.

Coconut oil

Unrefined coconut oil is made from the dried kernels of coconuts. It's naturally soothing to inflamed skin and is also naturally antifungal and antibacterial, which helps skin to heal faster. Its fatty acid profile makes it ultra-hydrating to the skin. Coconut oil has a smooth, slippery texture and has a little bit of a greasy feel – but this helps it to soothe irritated skin! Unrefined, raw coconut oil has a more medicinal effect as its fats and compounds are still intact.

Camellia seed oil

The Camellia oil, also known as tea seed oil, is an edible, pale amber-green fixed oil with a sweet, herbal aroma.

This oil offers many therapeutic and healing properties:
- antioxidant qualities and resists rancidity.
- anti-aging effects and protects the skin from free radical damage, all thanks to the high number antioxidants present in it.

Camellia seed oil is an amazing moisturizer for the skin because it contains high oleic acid omega 9 content.

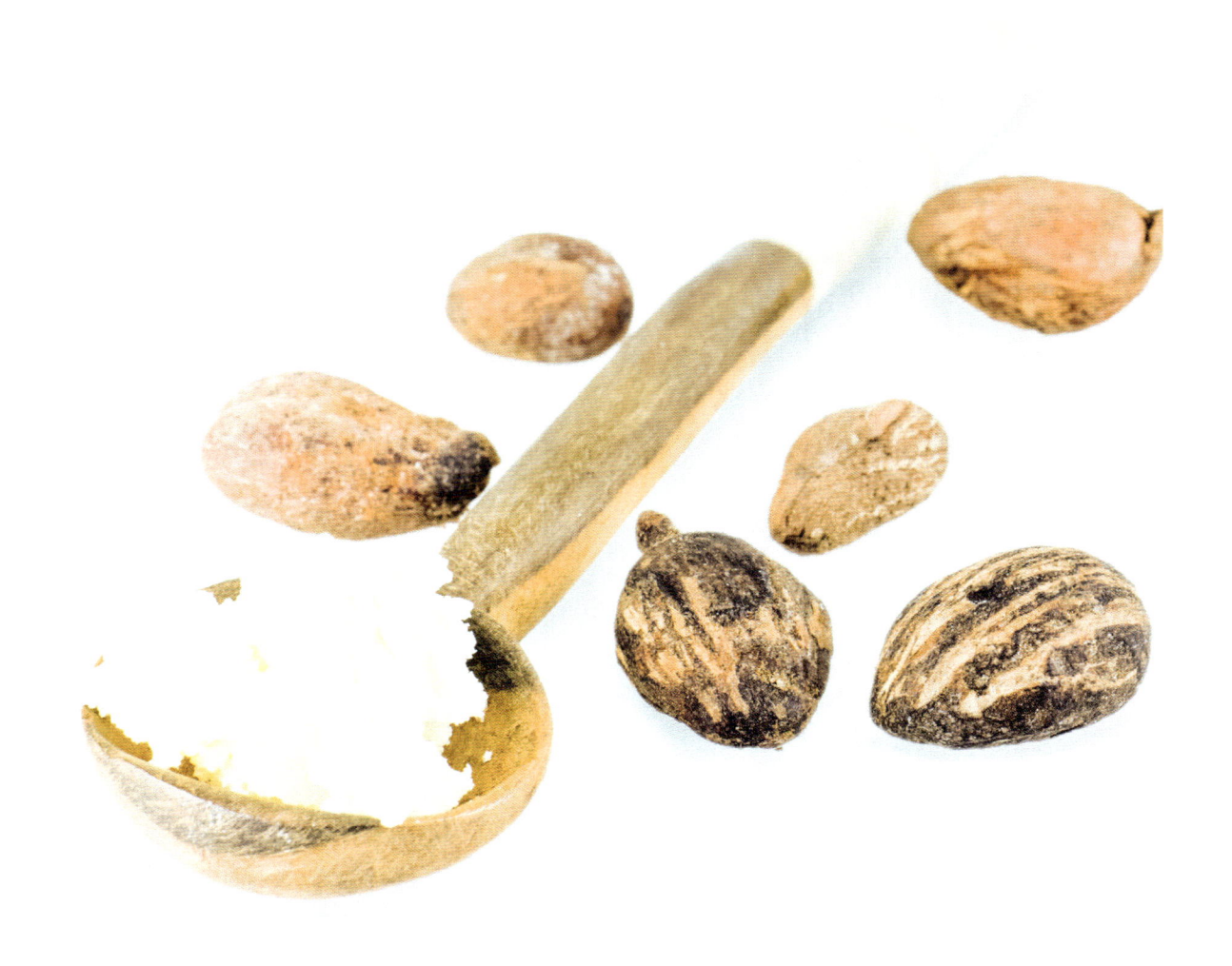

BUTTERS

THE ESSENTIALS

Shea butter
Shea butter adds a richness to this homemade face cream with its thick, creamy texture. It's made from the nut of the African shea tree. It has a soothing effect on the skin. It provides an added boost of Vitamin E and fatty acids, enabling it to nourish the skin and fight signs of aging as well.

Cocoa butter
Cocoa butter is made from cocoa beans and is richer, heavier butter that packs a lot of moisturizing and nourishing benefits. It is high in phytochemicals that have anti-aging properties, and it may even help to improve blood flow to the skin, giving you a natural glow!

If you prefer not to have a slight cocoa or chocolate smell, then use refined (deodorized) cocoa butter. I personally do not mind this sweet smell!

Mango butter
Mango butter is made from mango fruit tree seeds and is high in vitamins A and E, which help it to nourish and repair skin. It has a rich, luxurious texture, but is medium-speed absorbing oil, which means it penetrates the skin fairly well. Make sure that you are purchasing 100% pure mango butter that has not been blended with any other additives.

Ucuuba butter
Ucuuba butter is a rare seed butter made from the ucuuba plant of South America. The plant is also known as baboonwood and wild nutmeg. It is most prominent in the Amazon river basin, but is also found throughout the wetlands of Central and South America.

This uccuba butter is brown and has a specific sweet yet nutty smell. It is made from the seeds of this versatile plant can be used on both the skin and hair.

It's superpower, however, lies in its anti-inflammatory effect, which can be very healing for a variety of skin conditions. It is also high in lauric acid and palmitic acid, both of which are important for healthy cell development, making the balm ideal for restoring skin tone and texture.

Ucuuba butter is also high in Vitamin C, which helps to reverse skin damage and is a powerful anti-aging agent, and Vitamin A, also known as retinol. Retinol is commonly used in top-of-the-line skincare products to treat acne, fine lines, and other signs of aging.

Kokum butter
Kokum butter is from India. It is high in vitamin A and rich in lauric, myristic and oleic acids. It is a light, protective butter that both moisturizes and protects the skin without feeling greasy. Kokum has antibacterial, anti-inflammatory, and antioxidant properties making it an ideal moisturizer for oily or acne prone skin. It is also excellent for making a homemade anti-aging product.

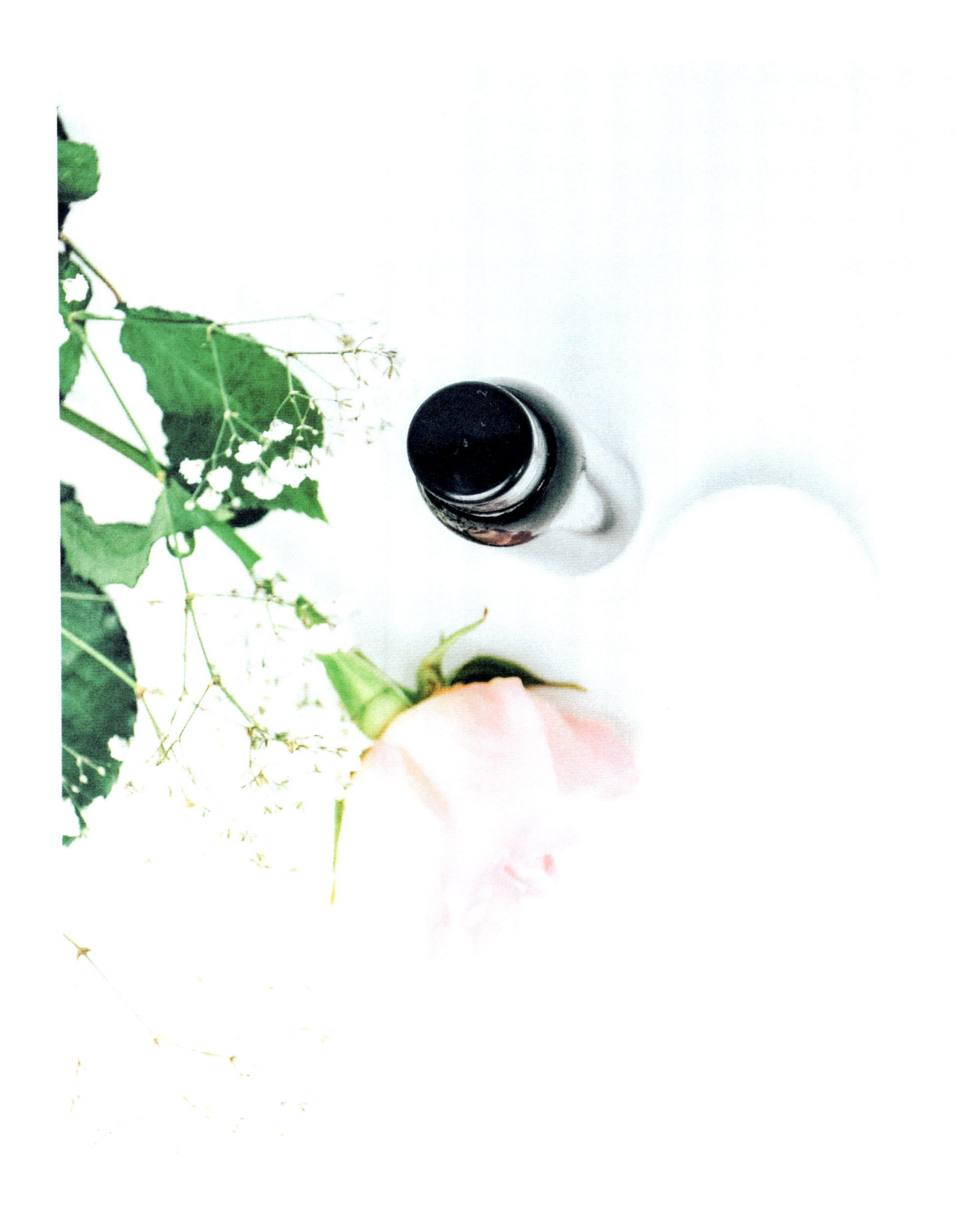

HYDROSOLS AND FLOWER WATER

THE ESSENTIALS

Orange blossom hydrosol

The orange blossom hydrosol is the result of extracting essence out of orange blossoms through the distillation process. It is the water that evaporates and not the essential oil. It's a commonly used ingredient for natural perfumes, toners, and aftershave even from the olden days. It slows down the aging of the skin and is safe for sensitive and delicate skin types, perfect to add in a DIY face moisturizer.

Orange blossom can be used for:
- Skin cleansing
- Skin exfoliation
- Treating acne
- Tightening the pores

Chamomile hydrosol

Chamomile flower water or hydrosol is derived from chamomile flowers. It is naturally calming due to the types of naturally occurring esters and alcohols in the plant. Chamomile water is nourishing to the skin, anti-inflammatory and antiseptic – making it great for this eye makeup remover.

Rosewater or rose hydrosol

Extracted from roses through a steam distillation process, not only does rose water smell heavenly, but it also boasts a number of benefits. Full of antioxidants, it's one of the best remedies for alleviating sensitive skin problems, and soothing skin irritation and redness.

28 ORGANIC BEAUTY RECIPES BY EVE

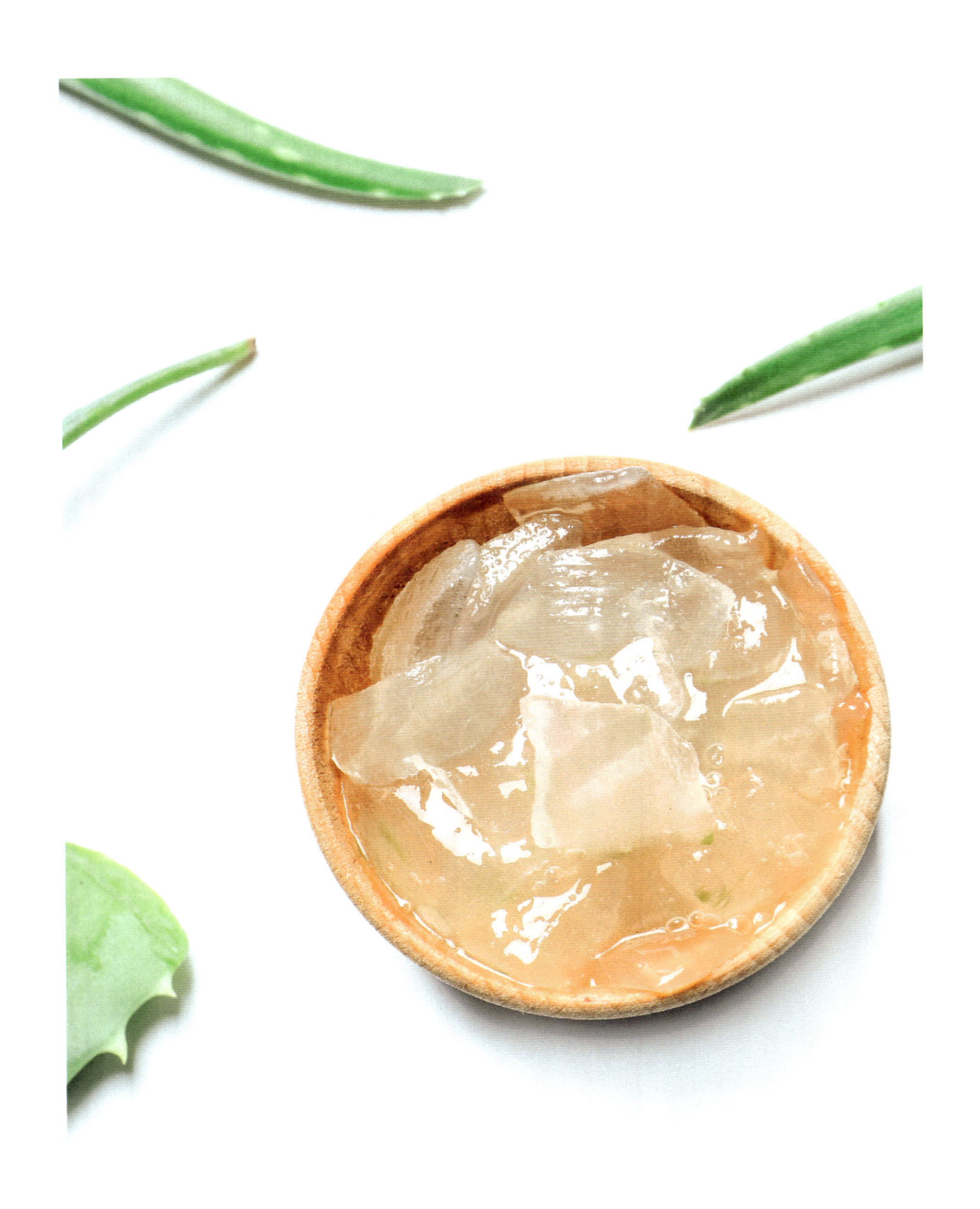

ALOE VERA

THE ESSENTIALS

I use aloe vera in some of my beauty care recipes as this plant is great for healing. Aloe vera is a species of succulent plant that grows in arid climates and is widely distributed in Africa, India and other arid areas. It is useful in the treatment of wound and burn healing, minor skin infections...

The best aloe vera gel you can find is from the fresh leaves but if do not live in a dry climate, you can buy aloe vera gel or juice online at any health food stores. Make sure you always buy organic aloe vera juice with 100% juice or gel with no preservatives. Unfortunately most manufacturers add preservatives as aloe vera spoils easily so be sure to read the labels. You must keep it refrigerated once the bottle is open.

My favorite aloe vera is Aloe Vera Juice Organic Whole Leaf with No Preservatives from Lily Of The Desert.

How to prepare aloe vera gel from fresh leaves

1. Choose aloe vera leaves that are large and mature, but still soft and succulent with plenty of moisture and gel inside. Avoid the small leaves as they will not contain enough gel.
2. Cut the leave from the base of the plant and let the yellow sap (called aloin) runs out of the leaves for a few minutes on a towel.
3. When the yellow sap is all gone, take a sharp knife and use it to remove the spiky edges from the leaves.
4. The leaves will have spiky edges to protect the plants from animals that also like the sweet gel inside the leaves.
5. Once the thorns have been removed, use the paring knife to peel one side of the leaf, so that you will have access to the gel.
6. Use a tea spoon to transfer the gel to a sterilized can.
7. Add a few drops of grapefruit extract to help with preservation.
8. Always keep the fresh aloe vera gel inside the fridge.

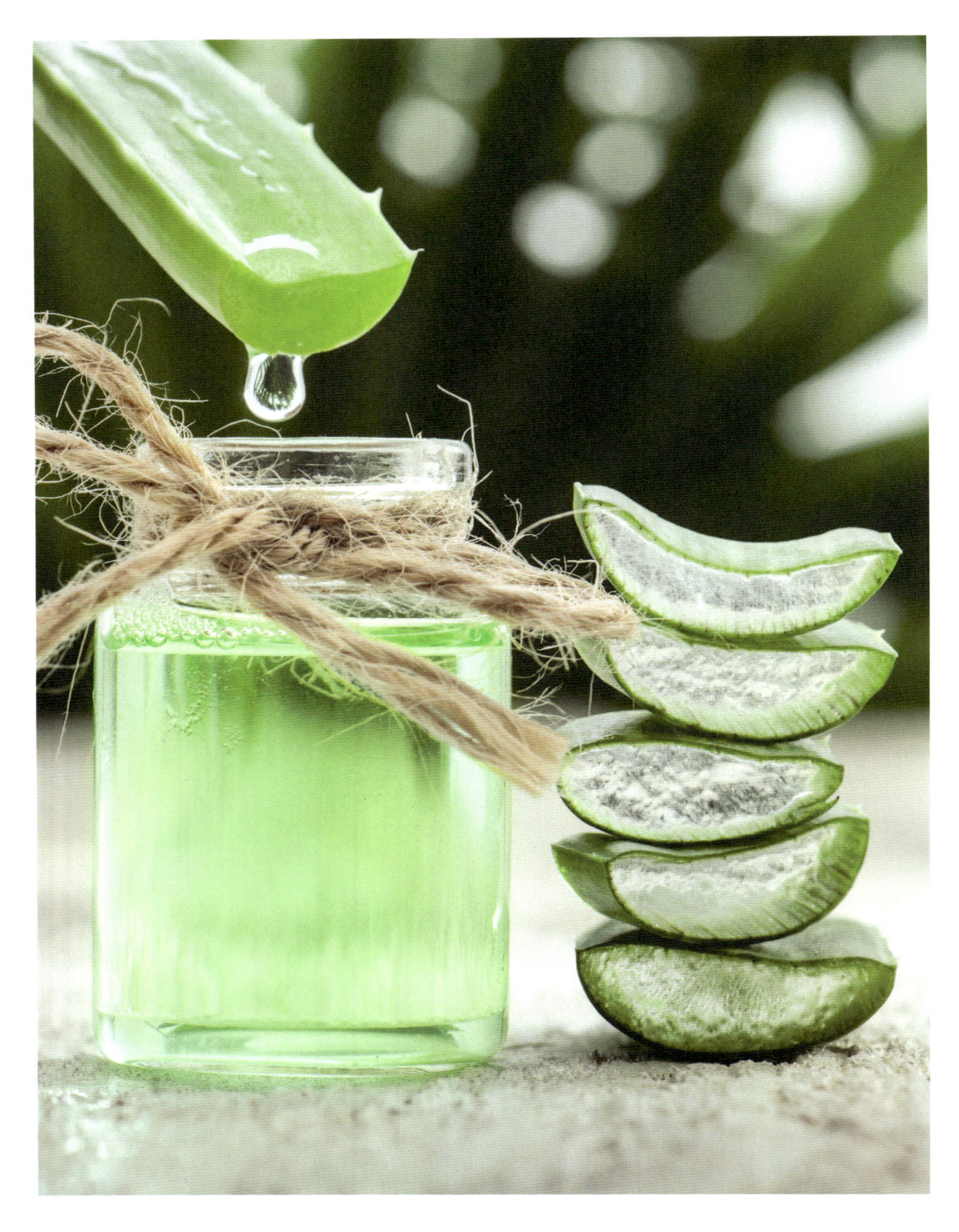

ALOE VERA HEALING CLEANSER AND AFTER SUN SOOTHER

THE ESSENTIALS

Aloe Vera is anti-inflammatory, antibacterial and helps heal wounds of all kinds. It is great to use on your face as a toner and healing agent for acne. It also works wonders if you apply on sunburns. Suitable for all skin type.

PREP TIME: 5 MINUTES

TOTAL TIME: 5 MINUTES

INGREDIENTS

- 1 cup of organic 100% Aloe vera gel
- 1/4 teaspooons of vitamin E
- 5 drops of lavender essential oil
- 3 drops of roman chamomile essential oil
- 25 drops of grapefruit seed extract as a natural preservative

INSTRUCTIONS

- Combine all ingredients in a dark coloured glass.
- Shake well before use and keep in the fridge.
- This can also be use on the body as an after sun soother.

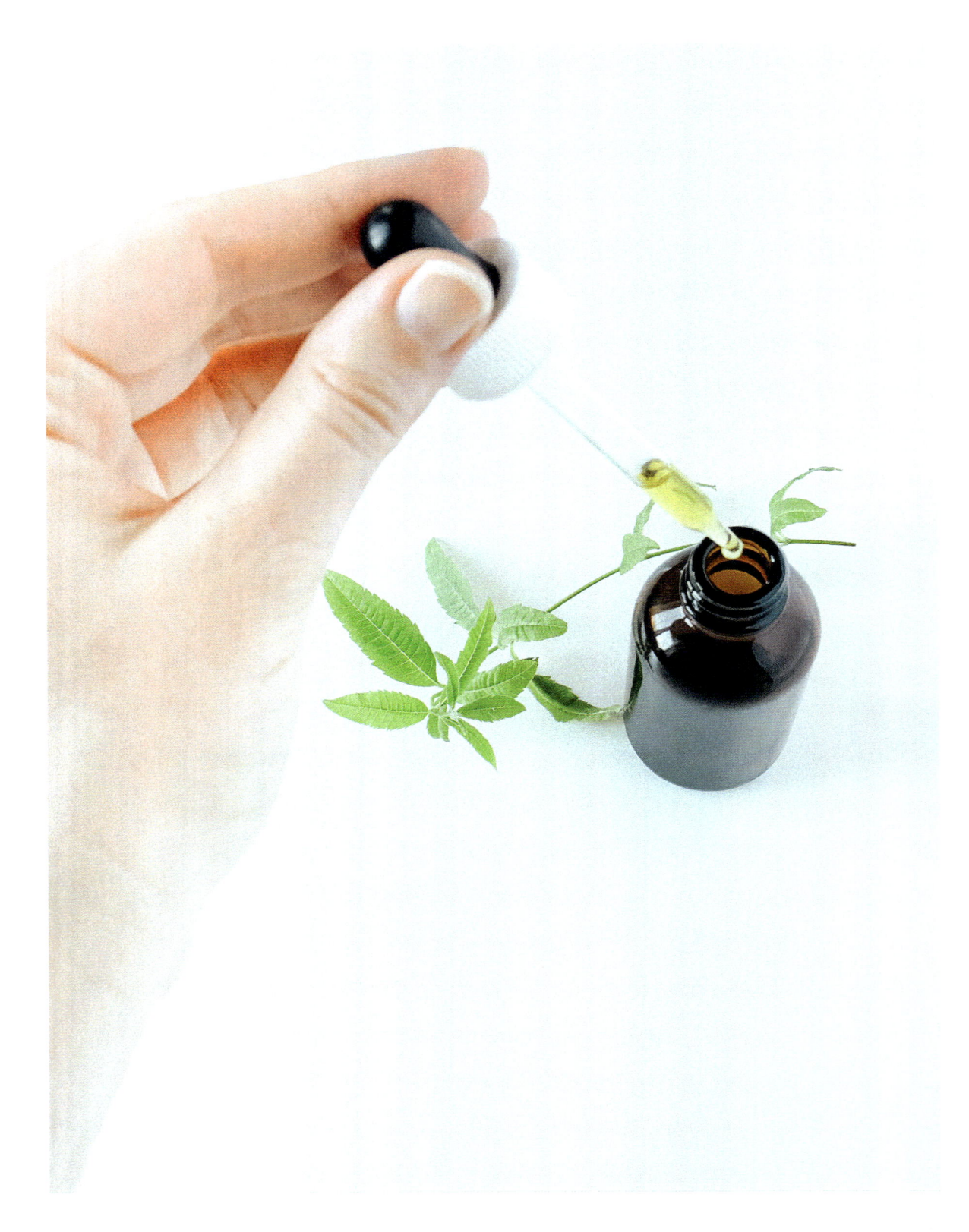

ESSENTIAL OILS

THE ESSENTIALS

You will find below my top 5 favorite essential oils that I use often in my recipes and are in my opinion must haves in your pantry!

Lavender essential oil
Lavender essential oil is made from the flowers of the lavender plant. It is also effective at visibly reducing redness in the skin. Lavender is grown all over the world, but some of the best lavender comes from Provence, France. Lavender essential oil can also help to reduce the formation and appearance of sunspots. I also use one drop before going to bed and it helps me with a restful deep sleep!

Roman Chamomile essential oil
Roman Chamomile essential oil is distilled from a particular type of chamomile, Roman chamomile, known in Latin as Anthemis nobilis. It is antiseptic, antibacterial, soothing and can even be used as a sedative – perfect for inflamed and painful sunburn.

Frankincense essential oil
Frankincense essential oil is a natural astringent that can kill germs and bacteria, and is also made from a type of plant. Frankincense comes from the resin of a tree native to the Middle East, and has long been used bot for its rich, pleasing scent and its medicinal properties.

Peppermint essential oil
Peppermint essential oil's amazing healing and soothing properties protect your lips from extensive damage while also soothing any irritation. It will provide a fresh and tingling sensation when used in homemade lip balms!

Rose Geranium essential oil
Geranium essential oil, is distilled from a rose-scented geranium flower and has natural antiseptic properties which make it ideal for treating inflammatory conditions like acne. It smells great and is especially soothing to the skin.

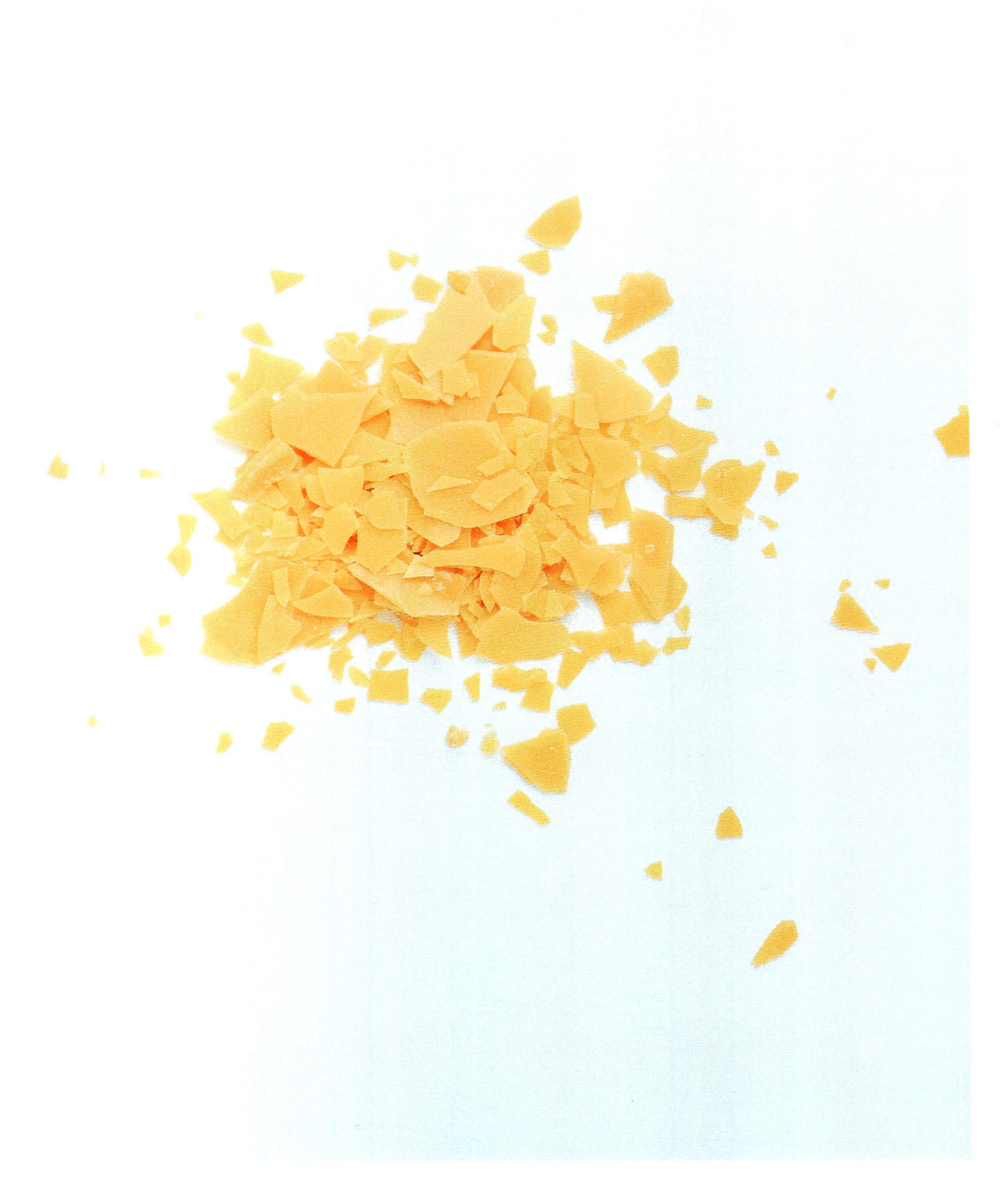

NATURAL EMULSIFIERS

THE ESSENTIALS

'Emulsifier' and 'emulsion' are words that get used a lot in DIY beauty products. Cosmetic companies use all sorts of chemical or synthetic emulsifiers, but the good news is that there are plenty of natural emulsifiers out there too! Here are my top 5 natural emulsifiers so you don't have to use chemicals ever again, beeswax, candelilla wax, carnauba wax, rice bran wax and organic liquid lecithin.

What is an emulsion?

This is simple process that blends oil and water and helps you to create a smooth consistency in your beauty products. An emulsion is a mixture of molecules that create a smooth blend of all the same size molecules. For instance, a lighter oil may have small molecules and a heavier butter may have large molecules. To mix them successfully, you will need an emulsifier. The emulsifier helps to bridge the small molecules and the larger molecules, resulting in molecules that are all the same size.

Beeswax

Beeswax is made from the honeycomb of bees and provides a natural protective barrier when applied to the skin. It is also an anti-inflammatory, moisturizing wax with a thick, tacky texture, which makes it a good stiffening agent in DIY beauty products. This is one of my favorite natural emulsifiers because it is very versatile. You can use it to create lip balm, lip gloss, salves, body butter, creams, massage bars, candles, wood polish and much more!

Melting point is 62 to 64 °C.

Carnauba Wax

Carnauba wax is an edible wax made from a Brazilian palm tree. It is one of the hardest natural waxes available and it provides a glossy finish in natural cosmetics. It is highly emollient, delivering moisture to the skin.

Melting point: 80-86 oC

Rice Bran Wax

Rice Bran Wax (Oryza Sativa) is a wax that can be used in lipstick, salves, body butter but also creams and lotion. This is a good alternative to use if you are vegan.

The melting point is 75/80C.

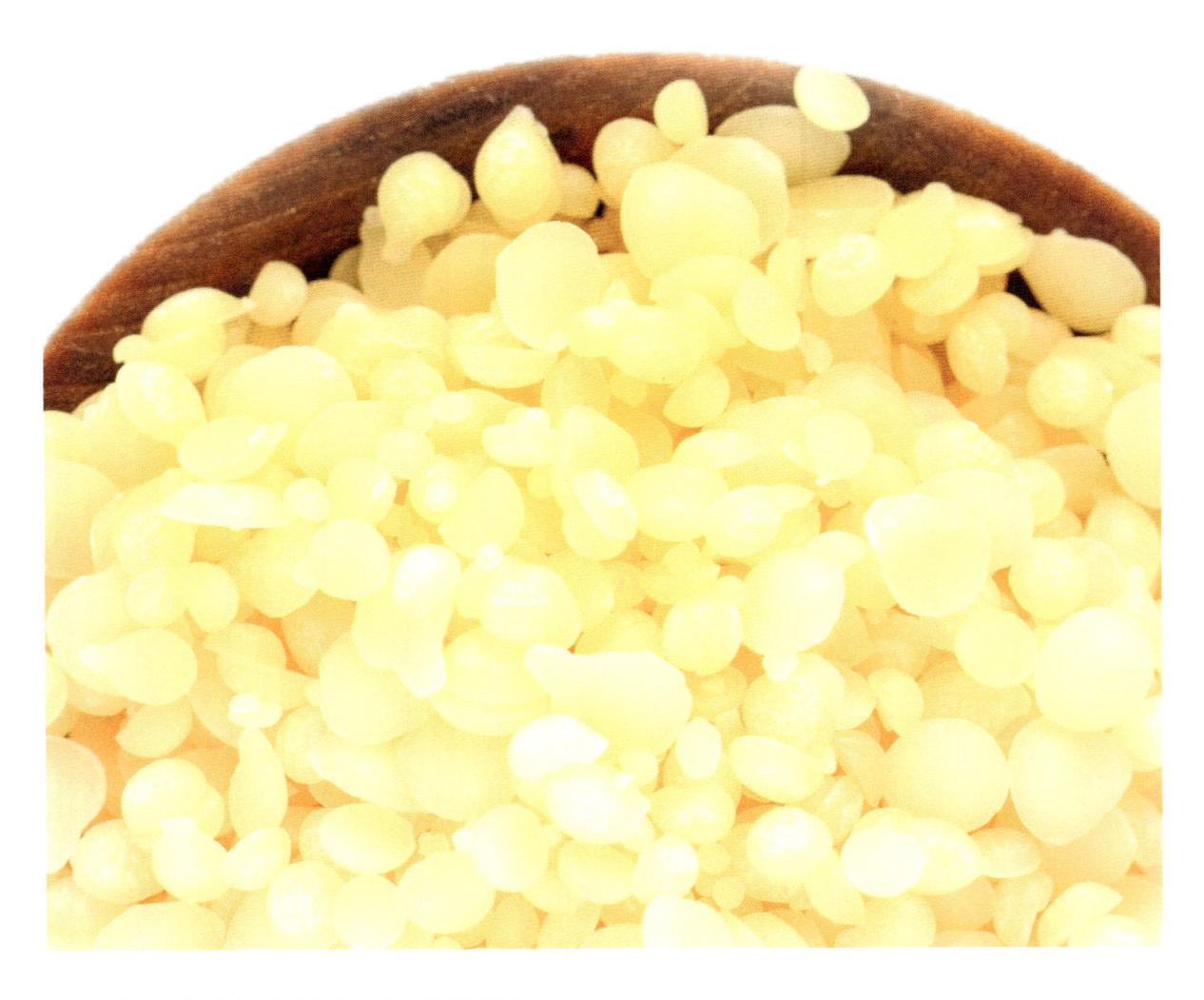

Liquid Lecithin

Liquid Lecithin is a naturally occurring fat found in both plants and animals. Lecithin is an emulsifier and restores skin health by reducing flakiness and dryness. It is also used as a thickener, stabilizer, mild preservative, moisturizer, and emollient in natural beauty products. The only thing I do not like about lecithin is that it comes from soybeans and is solvent extracted.

Naturally-derived emulsifier

Naturally derived emulsifiers means they are not 100% natural and are made in a lab, a good example is Emulsifying wax (e.g olive1000). They have a high melting point and can help to create an ultra-smooth cream.

Why you might choose to use a Naturally-derived emulsifier

I personally don't use emulsifiers that are made in a lab. They can, however, be useful if you want to make a liquid lotion that is not greasy. If you are looking to recreate the nongreasy texture of more conventional beauty products, using an naturally derived emulsifier is the way to go. Just keep in mind, your beauty product will NOT be 100% natural.

Can you make a cream or body butter without an emulsifier?

The answer may surprise you, but it is a 'yes'. And it is my favorite way of making a cream or body butter without any beeswax, or emulsifying wax.

Basically, if you use butter and a carrier oil and mix them very fast with a high speed blender, it will create a cream and even sometimes whipped body butter. Even though it is not a proper emulsion, the end result is still a body cream.

How to make a basic cream or lotion using an emulsifier

To make a cream or lotion with an emulsifier, you will need to:

1 Melt down the natural wax with your other ingredients (oil, butter, hydrosol)

2 Blend thoroughly until you create a cream or lotion.

Be sure to pay attention to the ratios your specific recipe calls for. If you use too much water content (hydrosol), the cream will separate.

If you are inventing your own recipe using a natural emulsifier, you typically want to use between 5% to 10% of the emulsifier.

38 ORGANIC BEAUTY RECIPES BY EVE

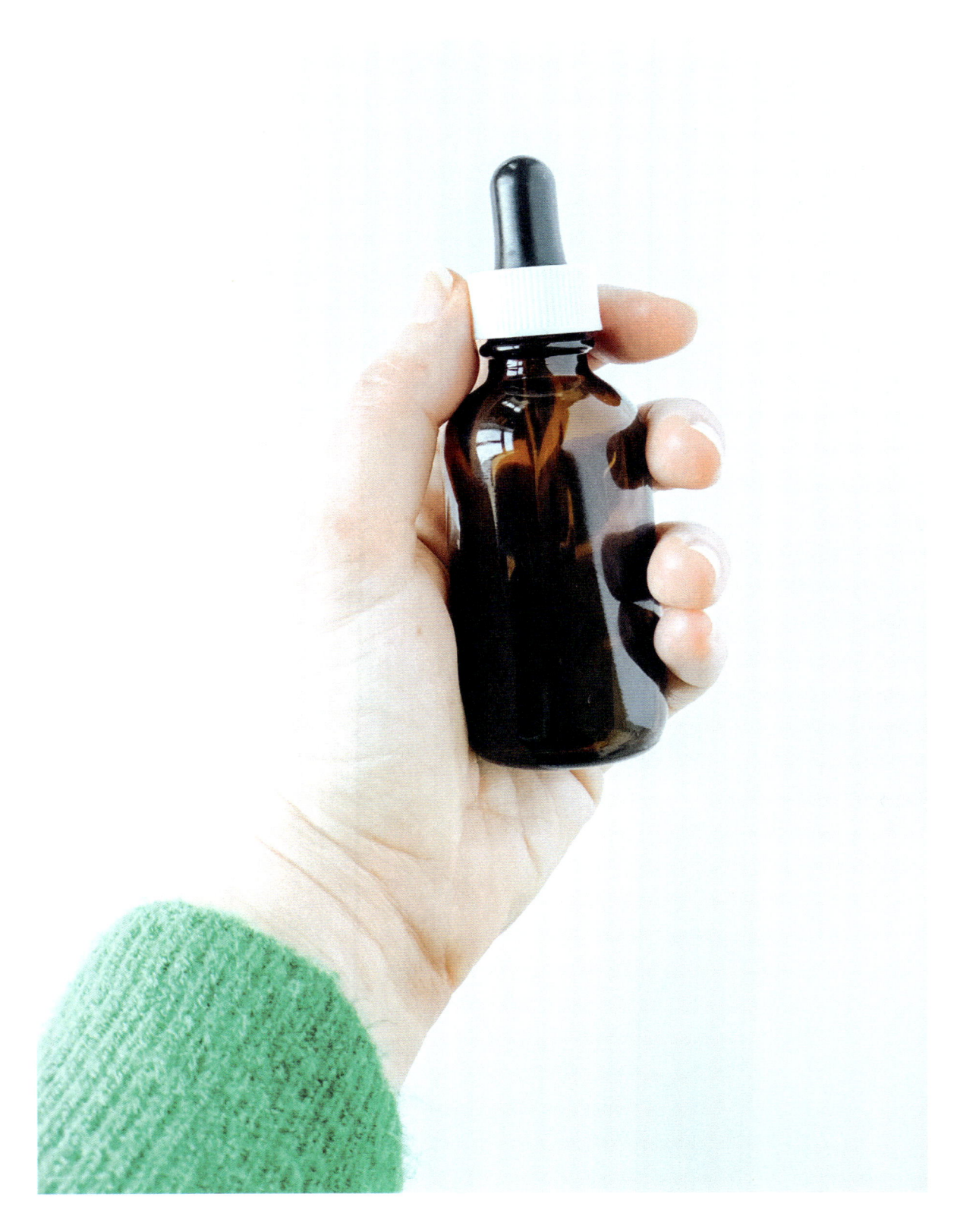

NATURAL PRESERVATIVES

THE ESSENTIALS

*M*y top 3 natural preservatives for DIY beauty products are Rosemary oil extract, Grapefruit seed extract and Essential oils.

Keeping your homemade body products fresh is a common concern – after all, one of the things you are trying to avoid when switching to DIY beauty products is adding synthetics preservatives or any sorts of chemicals.

That would defeat the purpose of making natural and organic DIY products!

Fortunately, there are a number of natural preservatives that you can use in your homemade body products. There are also several tips you can use to reduce your need for DIY beauty products, which I will share below.

When to use Natural Preservatives in your homemade beauty products?

The rule of thumb is that you do not need to add preservatives to your DIY beauty products unless there is water content (such as aloe vera, hydrosol or mineral water).

When you make lip balms or body butter with only oils as the only ingredients, the shelve life is pretty much as long as the butter or oils themselves meaning from 6 to 18 months. There is no need to add a preservative for lip balms and body butter, as long as you do not add water content.

I recommend making new small batches of cream every month or so will also allow you to modify your recipes according to the season and to your skin needs.

If you sterilize (boil in water for 20 minutes, all instrument and use clean hands when touching creams, the shelve life of a cream or lotion with water with natural preservatives can be up to 1 month.

Just use common sense and smell or look for any signs that your lotion has become rancid or spoiled.

Introducing water (or aloe vera, and hydrosols) makes things go rancid or bad more quickly, this is why you have to make creams or lotions that include a water content in small batches and should use them up within a short period of time.

When making creams or lotions with water content, you can add the following natural preservatives to help extend the shelf life.

You can also keep your creams in the fridge so they last longer.

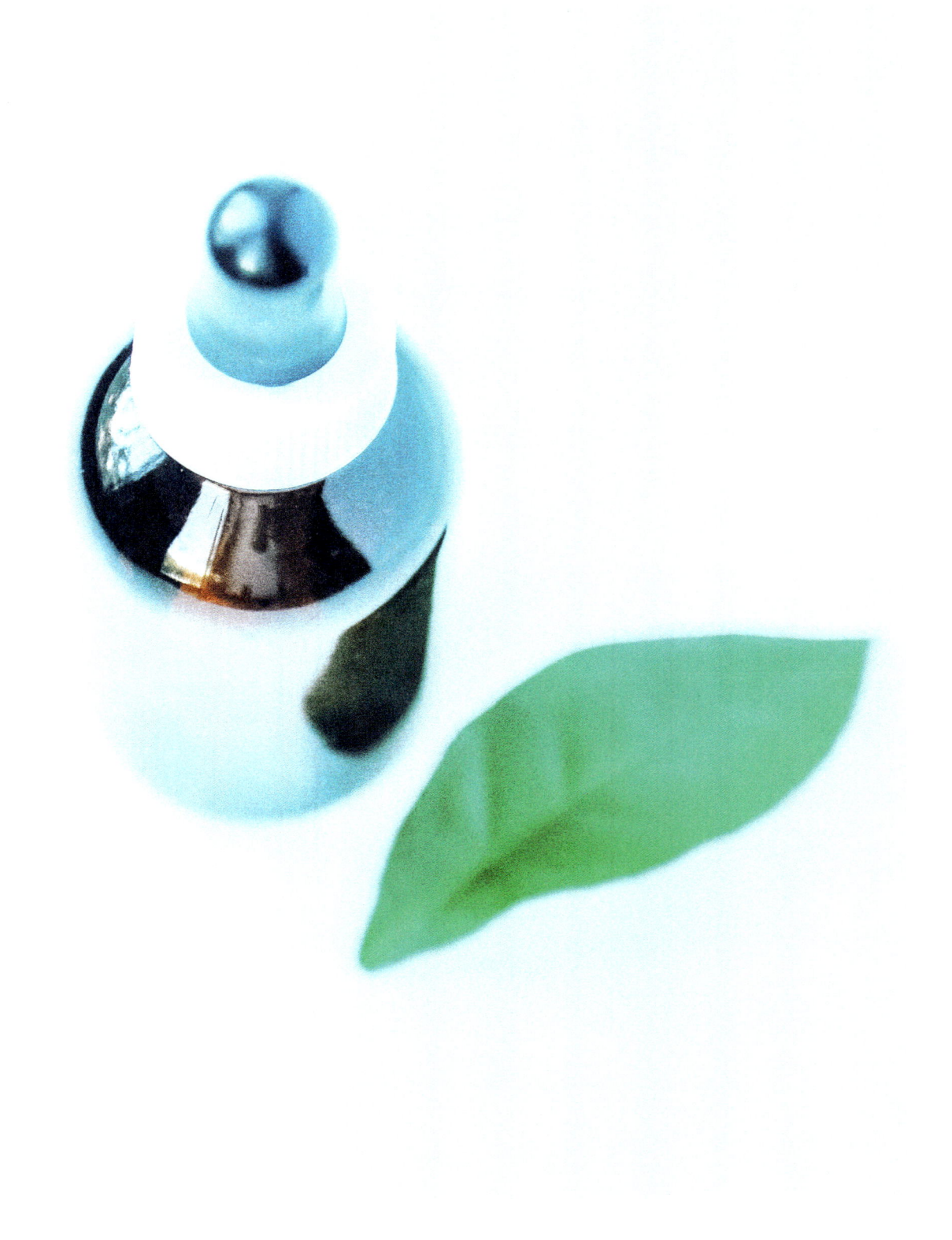

TOP 3 NATURAL PRESERVATIVES IN DIY BEAUTY

THE ESSENTIALS

Antioxidants
These are typically derived from food-sources and come in the form of thick gel-like oil. You only need a little bit to extend the shelf life of your body products. These also have naturally anti-aging benefits to the skin.

1

Rosemary oil extract
Rosemary oil extract is derived from the rosemary herb. It's naturally antiseptic and can help to protect skin from free radical damage, and is therefore anti-aging. It has a refreshing scent and is lighter textured oil.

Use in your formulation from 0.02% to 0.5% to extend the shelf life of your homemade product.

Anti-Microbials
They are naturally antibacterial agents that help to prevent the spread of bacteria in your product once it is made. Natural antimicrobials include liquids distilled from things like radish root. These help to prevent the spread of bacteria, mold or yeast.

2

Grapefruit seed extract
Grapefruit seed extract is another natural anti-microbial that also has high antioxidant content so that it packs a double punch. It may be lightly scented of citrus and has a very light consistency.

Use it 0.5 to 1% to preserve your products. Wear gloves while handling Grapefruit Seed Extracts it can be irritating to the skin undiluted.

3

Essential oils
Essential oils like lavender, tea tree, eucalyptus, and peppermint are all also naturally antibacterial. They can help to impart a scent to your body product and typically also have other beneficial properties such as being anti-inflammatory. They also have a very light, liquid consistency and of course amazing scent in addition to other health benefits.
Common dilution of essential oils is between 1% to 2% in your homemade products.

Why I don't use chemical preservatives
There are some preservatives on the market that can be added to your DIY beauty products, however, I do not recommend them. Here is why:

Germaben II is a broad spectrum preservative and is often used in deodorants, ammoniated dentifrices, mouthwashes, hair colorings, hand creams, lotions, shampoos.

While it may be effective, it is full of parabens that disrupt the endocrine system and may be carcinogenic. It contains DIAZOLIDINYL UREA which is "an antimicrobial preservative that works by forming formaldehyde in cosmetic products. People exposed to such formaldehyde-releasing ingredients may develop a formaldehyde allergy or an allergy to the ingredient itself. In the U.S. approximately 20% of cosmetics and personal care products contain a formaldehyde-releaser and the frequency of contact allergy to these ingredients is much higher among Americans compared to studies in Europe."

There is strong evidence of Human skin toxicant or allergen. You can read more about it on skin deep.

Liquid Germall Plus is another synthetic preservative. It is paraben free, but it utilizes chemicals like propylene glycol and iodopropynyl butylcarbamate, both of which are skin irritants that have been linked to liver toxicity. Liquid Germall Plus is banned for use in body products in the European Union.

How to make sure your homemade beauty products don't spoil?

Aside from using natural preservatives, you need to ensure you are following really good hygiene and a clean environment when making DIY body products.

Make sure you follow these tips to ensure your DIY beauty products last longer:
- Make small batches
- Sanitize all utensils and containers
- Use clean gloves when making the products
- Avoid direct sunlight and UV rays, oxygen, heat, moisture
- Use natural preservatives when there is water content (aloe vera, mineral water…)
- Use clean and dry hands when using the product.

The controversial debate over DIY and preservatives

Marketing and big beauty and pharma companies try to scare us away from making our own products because it is to their advantage that we buy their products instead.

Beauty companies need preservatives due to mass production and the fact that their products often sit on shelves for long periods of time, 2 to 10 years or more. You can avoid this by making your own beauty products.

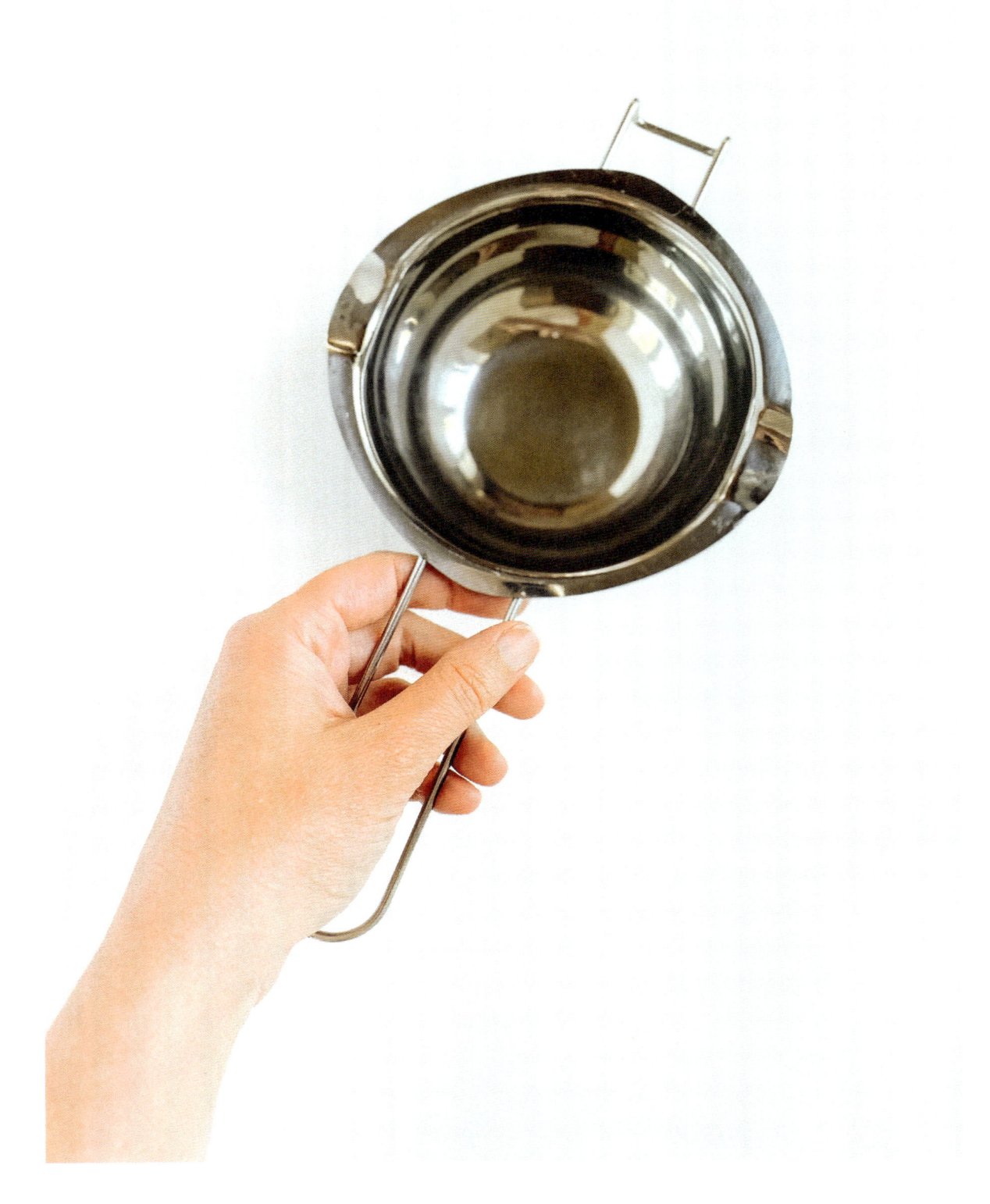

EQUIPMENT TO GET STARTED

THE ESSENTIALS

While you may have some of these items in your kitchen already, it's best to have equipment only reserved for your DIY beauty products.

Because of cross-contamination and for hygiene purposes, keep those utensils sterile or as clean as possible to avoid bacteria getting into your homemade products.

Plus, having the right equipment on hand will ensure that you can make any recipe you want to – from lip balms to body lotions.

My top 5 basic Equipment for DIY Beauty Products

1
Electric stick blender and hand whisk
This is a super versatile combination package that gives you a stick blender and hand whisk all in one. So many DIY beauty products require a powerful blender to thoroughly mix the ingredients. Nobody wants to apply lumpy lotion, right?

The stick blender and hand whisk do a beautiful job without requiring you to pour your recipe into a conventional blender, avoiding creating a bigger mess.

2
Hand whisk
Not all recipes need the power of an electric hand whisk – so you'll want to keep a good hand whisk around as well. This one has a comfortable rubber grip that keeps you from slipping but enables the dexterity to thoroughly blend your formulas. The stainless steel whisk can be used in heated recipes and is super easy to clean!

3
Protective gloves
If you want your DIY beauty products to last, they need to be made in a sterile environment as much as possible. This helps to reduce spoilage in the absence of preservatives – even though many DIY ingredients like some essential oils are naturally antibacterial, this extra step helps!

This also helps keep your skin from coming into contact with concentrated ingredients that you want to avoid. Nitrile gloves are the best because they allow you a sensitive but durable grip, and unlike latex gloves, they do not leave behind any powder or residue. You get many gloves in a box, making this an affordable option as well.

4
Double boiler
A double boiler is a must-have for many DIY beauty recipes. This will enable you to melt the butter down to liquid in order to blend them with other ingredients without burning them, for example. This Neeshow double boiler is made of stainless steel, so it can be used with high heat – and is also rust and stain resistant, and easy to clean! The best feature is the spouts

on either side. These enable you to pour your melted ingredients into your mixing bowls without dripping or a huge mess!

5
Stainless Steel Measuring Cups and Spoons Combo Set

If you have made DIY beauty products before, you know that precision is key!

Steer clear of plastic measuring cups or spoons and opt for stainless steel versions that are less corrosive and can handle a variety of materials at different temperatures. I love this set because the measuring cups nest for easy storage – having multiple cups instead of a single 2 cup with measuring marks also means less washing between uses.

The measuring spoons are in the sizes most often used, so this set really gives you everything that you could need at a great price!

All in all, this would be an investment of $60 and will last for years.

48 ORGANIC BEAUTY RECIPES BY EVE

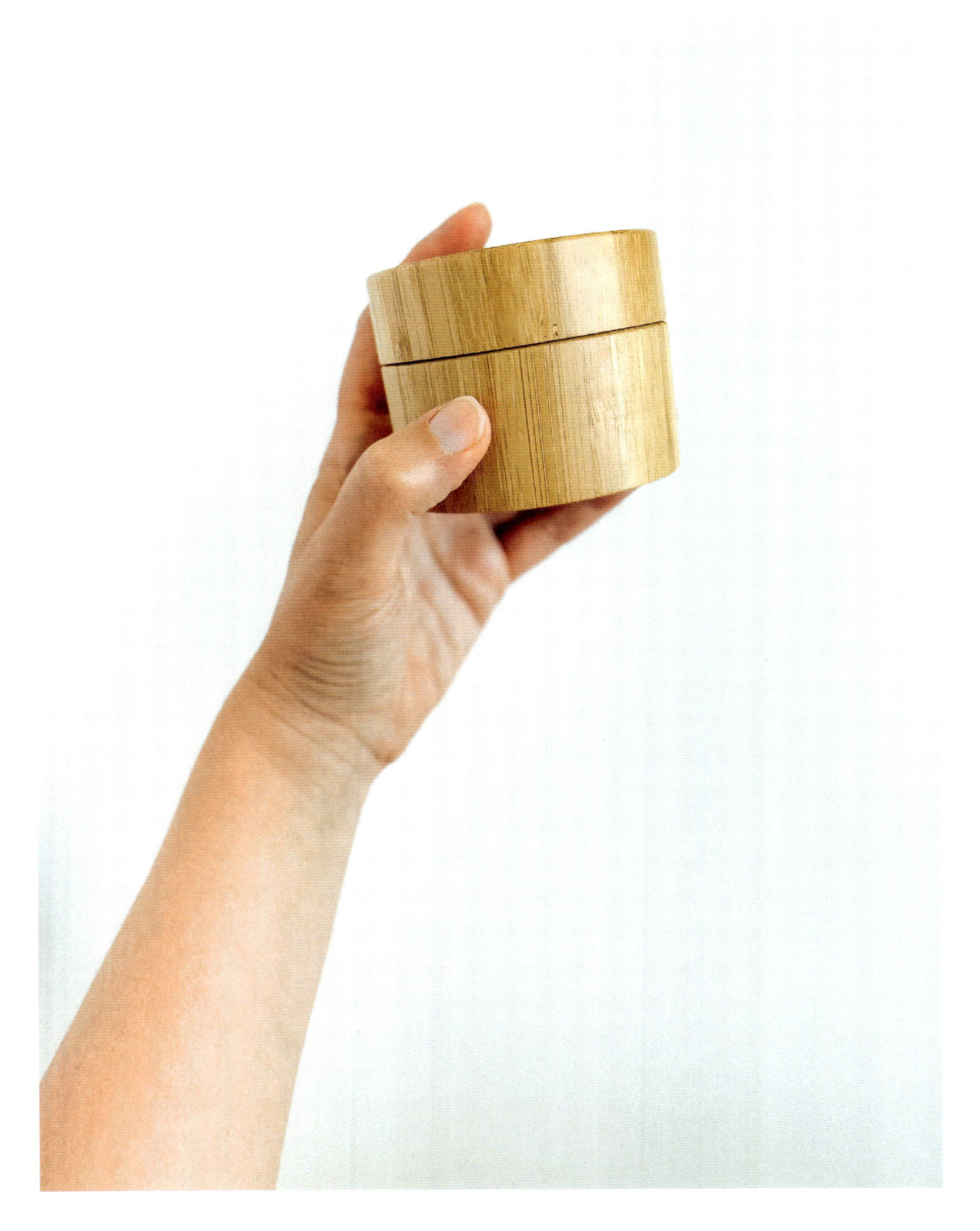

CONTAINERS

THE ESSENTIALS

The best place to find containers for homemade beauty products is on amazon.com

Body butter and creams

You can opt for plastic or glass jars for your homemade body butter, even mason jars can do the trick!

My preference is amber or cobalt blue glass containers. While there is a little more expensive than plastic, they last longer and are much better for the environment and for the product. If you choose plastic, make sure there is no BPA.

Another cheap option for container is round aluminium tins that are cost efficient and lighter than glass jars. They are great for travel!

Make sure the glass jar you use are made of high quality, food-safe glass and acrylic, BPA and lead free. If the glass is tinted, the bottles should be 100% tinted glass, never painted.

It is the best way to protect essential oils from UV since essential oils are photosensitive.

Here are my top choices for containers for homemade beauty products such as body butter or creams below:
- Cobalt Blue 1oz & 2oz Glass Straight Sided Jars
- 10ML High Quality Green Frosted Container Jars
- Silver Metal Steel Tins

Containers for Essential Oil blends or perfumes

You can use amber glass roll on bottles to keep you essential oil perfume oil. It makes a great gift and is perfect to travel or fit in your purse.

There is also some twisted look roll on perfume bottles available on the market. Some comes with silver or gold caps depending on your taste.

If you want to keep essential oil already blended, the best choice is to use cobalt or amber glass bottle with a glass eye dropper. Never use plastic to keep essential oils as they are corrosive and will eat the plastic eventually.

It's also important to use colored glass to preserve essential oils from losing their properties and health benefits as they get damaged from UV light.

50   ORGANIC BEAUTY RECIPES BY EVE

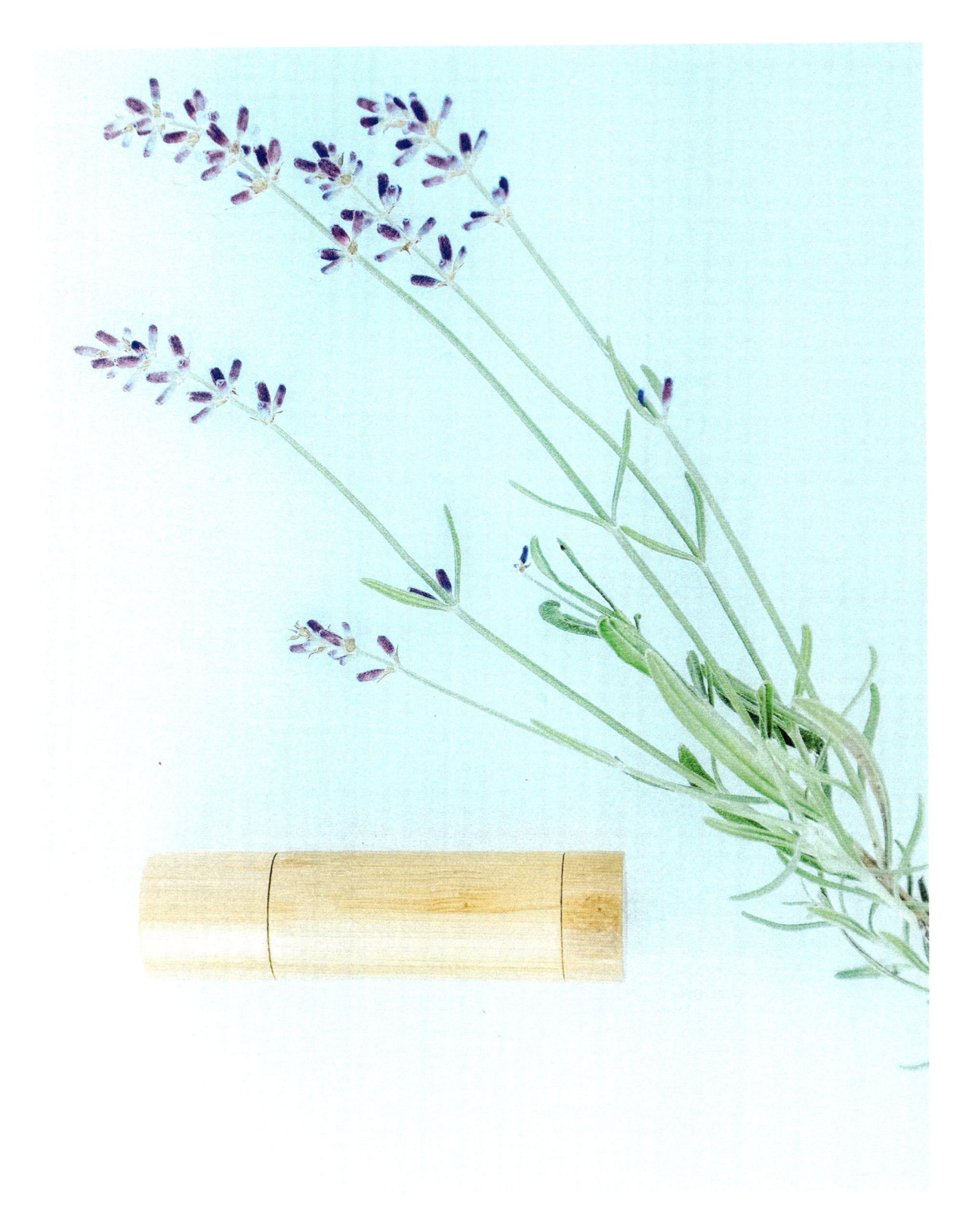

If you are working with aromatherapy, for mist spray, the best choice of container is refillable blue glass bottle with a fine mist dispenser.

Here are my recommended containers for essential oils blend:
- 1oz Amber Glass Bottles for Essential Oils with Glass Eye Dropper
- 4oz Empty Blue Glass Spray Misters
- All in one aromatherapy kit with spray bottle, rool one, pipettes, etc…
- 10 ml blue Glass roll on bottles with stainless steel roller balls

Containers for serums
- Amber Glass Vial for Fragrances, Serums, Spritzes, Essential Oils with Orifice Reducer and Dropper Top

Containers for homemade Lip balms
Amongst containers for homemade beauty products, you will most likely need empty lip balm tubes. You can choose lip balm tubes or lip balm slide tins or even rounded lip balm.

Here are some of my recommended choices for lip balm containers:
- Test Tube rack – This will help you stay organize and not make a mess on your table, highly recommended!
- 50, Clear, Empty, 5 Gram Plastic Pot Jars, Cosmetic Containers
- 50 clear lip balm tube transparent containers
- purple 10ML High Quality Frosted Container Jars with Inner Liner

52   ORGANIC BEAUTY RECIPES BY EVE

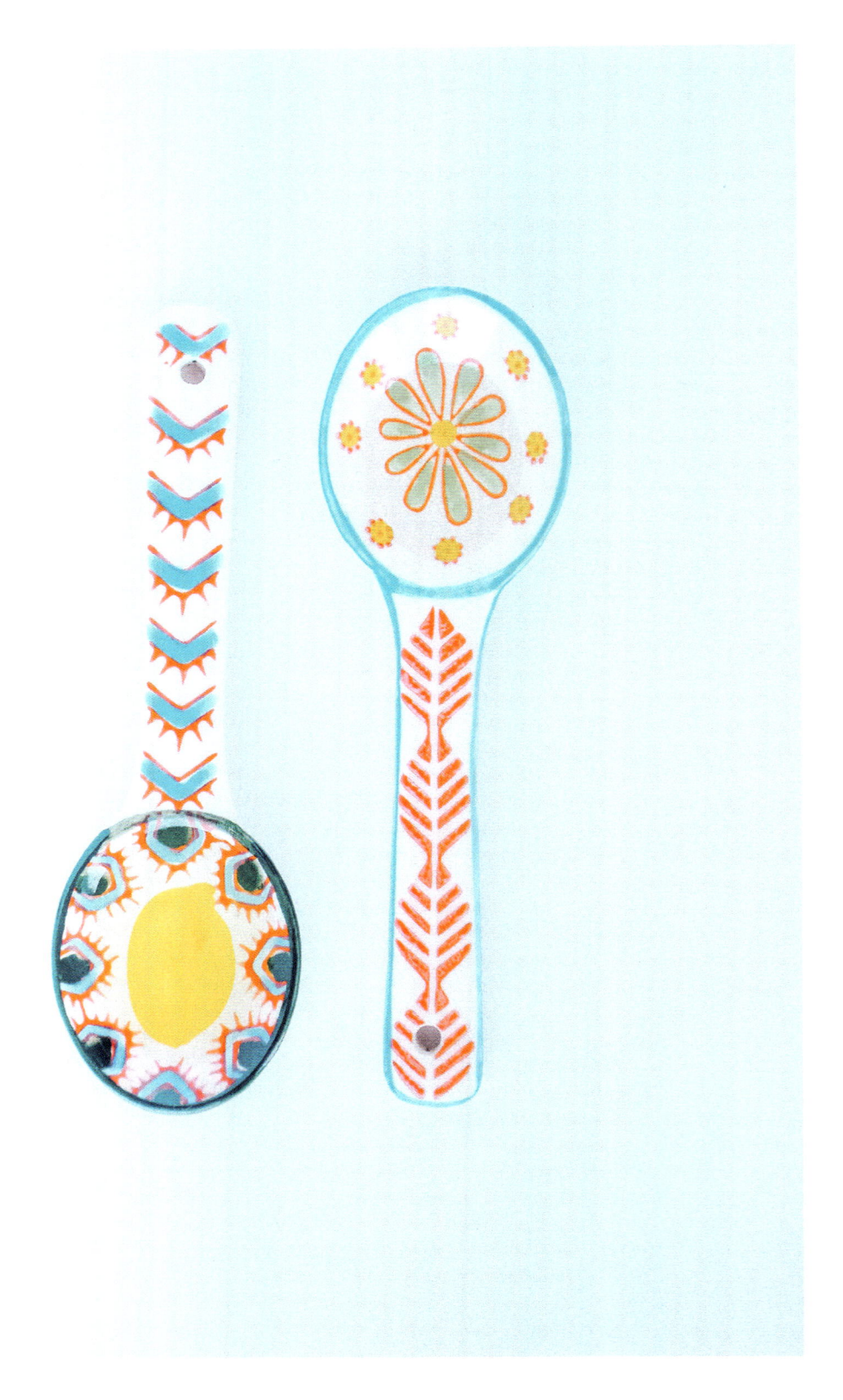

SUBSTITUTIONS IN DIY BEAUTY PRODUCTS

THE ESSENTIALS

The most frequently asked question I get is: can I replace this ingredient with another ingredient?

While most of the time, it changes the entire recipe, it is still possible to substitute one carrier oil for another. For example, you can replace is safflower oil instead of camellia seed oil.

Each carrier oil has its own properties when it comes to benefits to your skin, which is why you might choose one over another one. Or it may simply be a matter of what you have on hand. If you have purchased a lot of one ingredient, it makes sense that you would want to use it in as many recipes as possible.

A carrier oil is essentially the base oil in your beauty product. It is usually the most used ingredient in your recipe in proportion to the other ingredients, and it can make a big difference in terms of texture in your finished beauty product.

Common carrier oils include almond oil grapeseed oil and jojoba oil, but there are tons more out there! Each has its own benefits, nutrient composition, texture, melting point, and absorption rate.

TOP 3 RULES IN DIY BEAUTY INGREDIENTS SUBSTITUTION

For substitutions in DIY beauty products, you want to make sure that you use oil with similar properties to the one that you are replacing. Or, if you are making a marked change, be aware of the differences in the carrier oil you are selecting.

1

The speed of a carrier oil absorption in the skin

Not all oils blend into your skin the same way. Some have smaller molecules and absorb quickly, typically leaving little coating on the skin. Others have larger molecules – this gives them a luxurious, rich feel, but they absorb into the skin more slowly and may leave behind a faint and oily residue.

It's easy to feel the difference in absorption rates just by rubbing some of the carrier oil between your fingers. Note how long it takes to feel like it is gone, and if there is a noticeable coating on your skin afterward.

Fast absorbing carrier oils
These carrier oils absorb easily into the skin and are great if you want to create a non-greasy cream or face serum.
- grapeseed oil
- apricot kernel oil
- camellia seed oil

- safflower oil
- Rosehip oil
- Babassu oil
- Baobab Oil
- Hemp Seed Oil
- jojoba oil
- Moringa Oil
- Perilla Seed Oil

Average-speed absorbing carrier oils
These carrier oils absorb into the skin at average speed and can leave a slightly oily feeling on the skin.
- coconut oil
- argan oil
- sweet almond oil
- kukui nut
- cocoa butter
- sunflower oil
- Black Cumin Seed Oil
- Canola Oil
- Chia Seed Oil
- marula oil
- Meadowfoam
- Pomegranate Oil

Slow absorbing carrier oils
These carrier oils are to be used in a low proportion in your DIY beauty recipe formula. It is typically added to other carrier oils to enrich their protein and vitamin content.
- evening primrose oil
- avocado oil
- castor oil
- shea butter
- flax seed oil
- Carrot Carrier Oil
- olive oil
- Macamia Nut Oil
- neem oil
- oat oil

You will have the best results with substitutions in DIY beauty products if you swap carrier oils that are of a similar absorption rate. If you want to make a mixture thicker or lighter, you might substitute quick-absorbing oil for average rate oil for instance, but you may need to play with the ratio of the other ingredients.

2

The texture of the oil or butter
Each oil and butter has its own texture, which contributes to the formulation of the DIY beauty product. For lotions, it is easy to switch ingredients to produce a lighter or heavier textured cream. But, for other products, such as lip balms or lipsticks, the texture plays a huge role in giving the DIY beauty product its form, and you want to be especially careful with substitutions.

An oil may be liquid, soft or brittle.

Liquid oils
- Olive oil
- safflower oil
- argan oils

Soft Oils
- coconut oil
- shea butter
- mango butter

Brittle Oils
- Cocoa butter
- kukum butter
- illipe butter

Oils also have other properties and texture like being smooth, thick, or sticky. They can also have different smells so you need to take this into account when doing substitutions.

This will make a difference in your product so you need to pay attention to that as well!

3
The Melting point

The melting point is an important property of an oil when it comes to a recipe. Recipes are formulated around specific melting points.

So for the best substitution in your DIY beauty product, you want to choose a carrier oil with a similar melting point to the original one – otherwise, you will need to change the recipe too much to make a good end product. The melting point is also important for the application.

Oils with a higher melting point will not rub into the skin the same way as oils with a lower one. For instance, think of a lip balm: you want it to be firm to the touch but to melt into your skin on contact. Specific oils will help to achieve this effect.
- Coconut oil melts at 24°C (75°F)
- Shea butter at 38°C (100°F)
- Cocoa butter melts at 34°C

Looking at the above melting points, you can substitute Shea butter for cocoa butter if needed since they have similar melting temperatures.

You should avoid substituting coconut oil for Shea butter or cocoa butter as the texture as in the end beauty product would be different.

That being said, you can always experiment which is part of the fun of making DIY beauty products!

Tip **THE KEY TO SUBSTITUTIONS IN DIY BEAUTY PRODUCTS** is to be mindful of the specific properties of the carrier oil the recipe calls for and the one that you would like to use.

Using a carrier oil that is similar in texture, melting point, and absorption rate will give you a greater chance of success!

100%
HAND
MADE

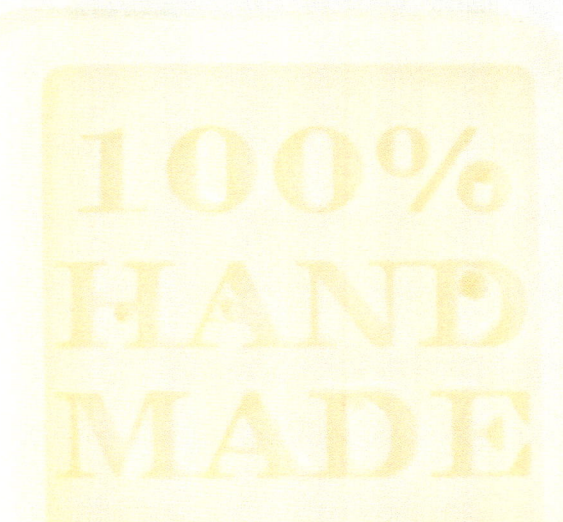

2 DIY BODY PRODUCTS

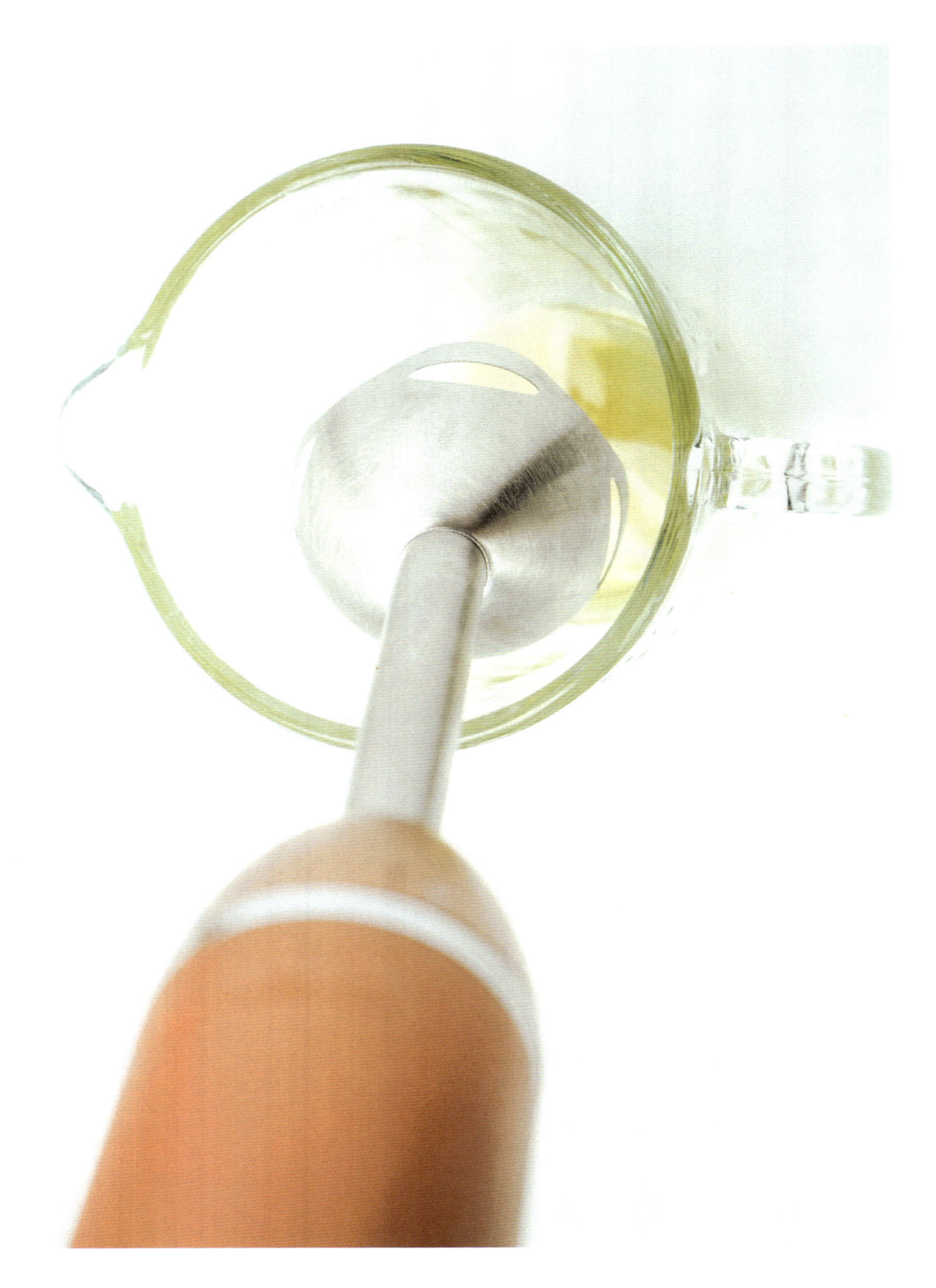

SHEA BODY BUTTER RECIPE WITH ONLY 2 INGREDIENTS

BODY BUTTER RECIPES

*I*f you are into a minimalist lifestyle or just getting started in DIY beauty, this shea body butter recipe is for you. You will learn how to make lotion with shea butter with only 2 main ingredients: organic shea butter and organic safflower oil and you can whip it in just 5 minutes.

You don't even need to heat it up nor use a double boiler for that matter. Yes, it's that simple!

PREP TIME: 5 MINUTES

TOTAL TIME: 5 MINUTES

MAKES: 100 ML / 3 OZ

INGREDIENTS

- 10 tablespoons of refined or raw shea butter
- 10 tablespoons of safflower oil
- 20 drops of lavender essential oil (Optional)
- a hand immersion mixer
- a glass recipient

INSTRUCTIONS

- Combine shea butter and safflower oil in a glass bowl.
- Start mixing the shea butter and safflower with a hand immersion mixer to make a shea butter lotion.
- Continue mixing until smooth, should take no more than 2 minutes to turn onto a cream.
- Add the essential oils if desired. (optional) Mix for a few seconds.
- Pour into a pretty container and slather the cream on your body, it will thank you!

Step by step how to make shea body butter

Step 1

Combine shea butter and safflower oil in a glass bowl.

Step 2

Start mixing the shea butter and safflower with a hand mixer.

Step 3

Continue mixing until smooth, should take no more than 2 minutes to turn into a cream. It will thicken as it settles.

Step 4

Pour into a pretty cream or lotion container and slather the cream on your body, it will thank you!

60   ORGANIC BEAUTY RECIPES BY EVE

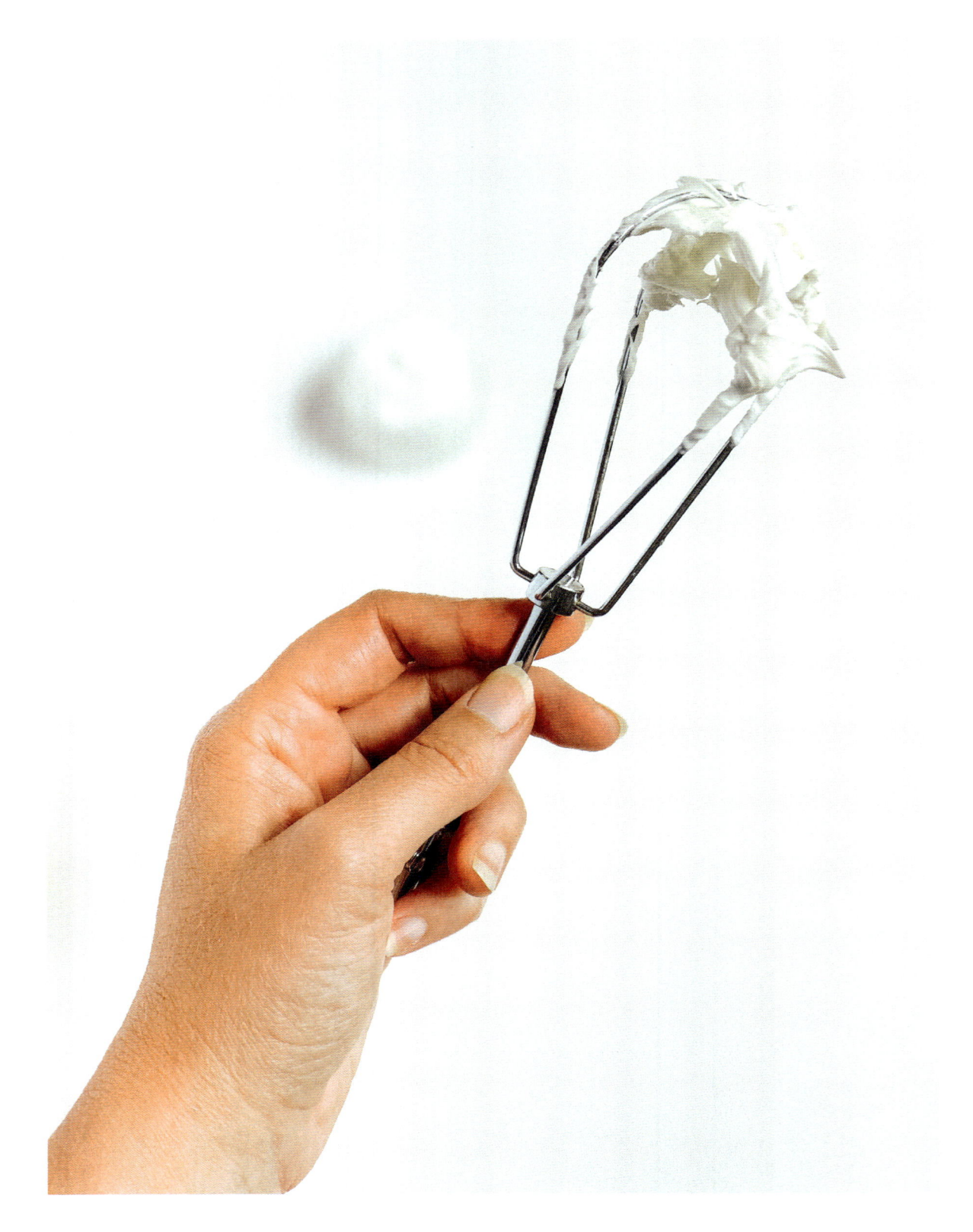

WHIPPED SHEA BODY BUTTER

BODY BUTTER RECIPES

This whipped shea body butter recipe is great if you are out of beeswax. It can be done in your kitchen for less than 20 minutes. It is an intense moisturizer and is wonderful for revitalizing dull or dry skin on the body.

PREP TIME: 15 MINUTES

TOTAL TIME: 15 MINUTES

MAKES: 300 ML / 10 OZ

INGREDIENTS

- 12 tablespoons of organic refined shea butter
- 2 tablespoons of organic mango butter
- 6 tablespoons of organic camelia seed oil
- Containers needed for this whipped body butter recipe:
- Glass Salve Containers
- Use a hand mixer like the one you would use for egg whites.

INSTRUCTIONS

- Put the shea and mango butter in a glass or metal bowl inside a pan filled with water on low heat so they starts melting slowly.
- Once melted add the camellia seed oil and mix well.
- Put in the freezer for 5 to 10 to 20 minutes until it has started to become a wax but is still soft and not completely frozen.
- Then take it out the freezer and start whipping with an electric whip (like a hand mixer you would use for egg white) on low speed.
- Make sure you wear an apron and that the bowl is deep enough so the butter does not start flying around everywhere in the kitchen!
- Begin whipping your mixture on low speed until it become foamy.
- Once the mixture is foamy, increase the speed to high until they become whipped to the desired stage.
- Add essential oils if desired at the end and whip for 1 min or less.
- Your butter will have a very fluffy and light consistency, like a nice whipped cream!

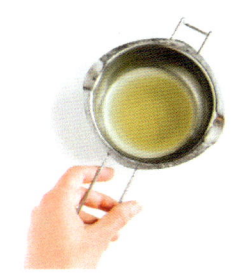

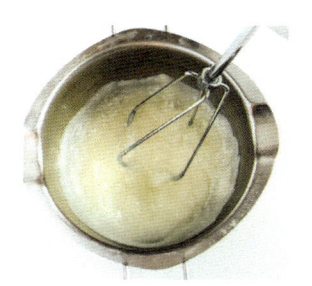

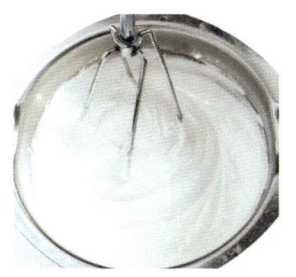

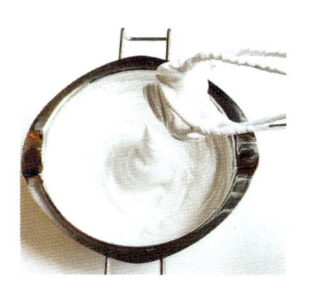

ORGANIC BEAUTY RECIPES BY EVE

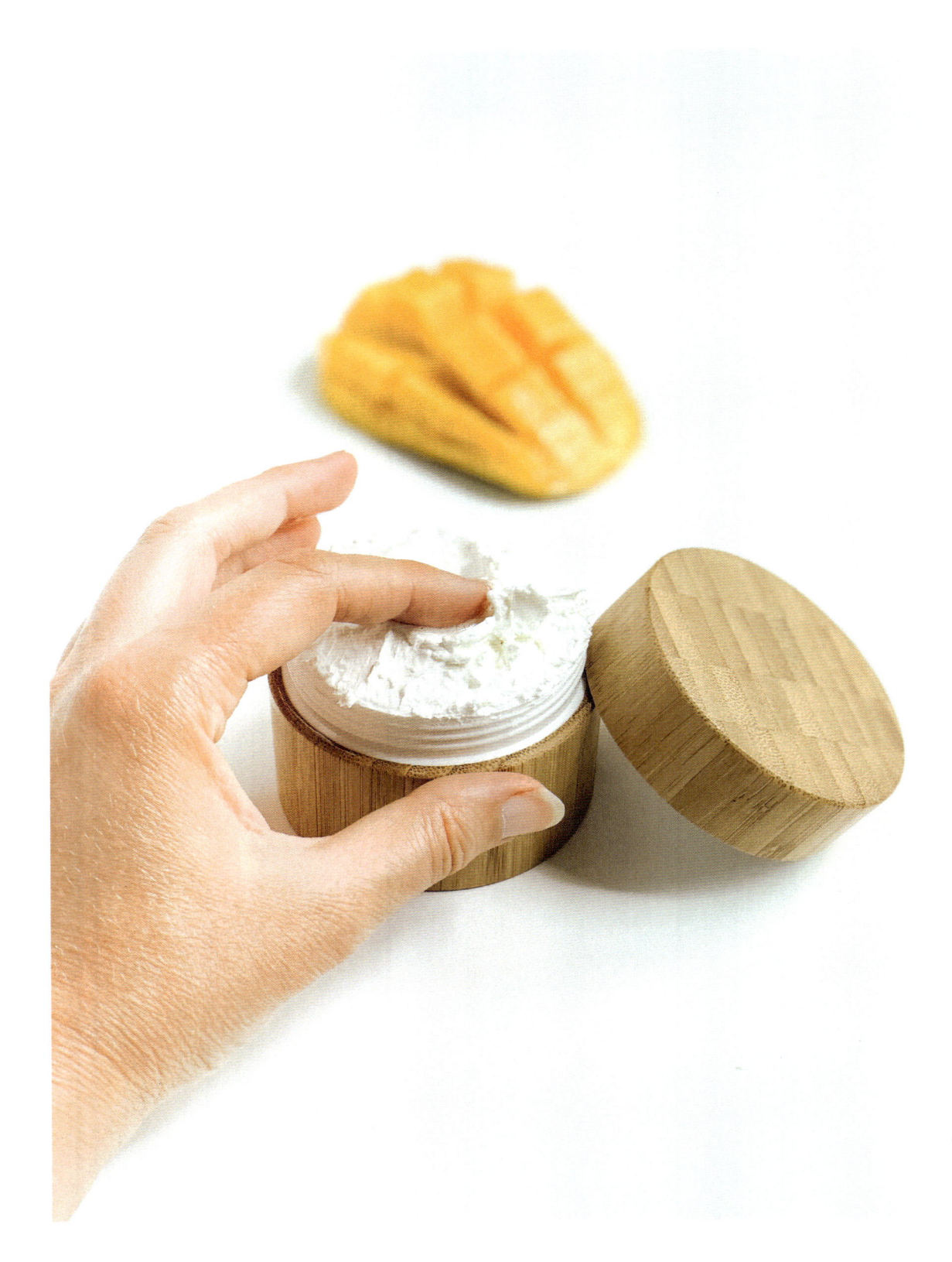

MANGO BODY BUTTER

BODY BUTTER RECIPES

*O*nce you have made my mango body butter recipe below, I think you will have trouble making anything else... This mango body butter melts right away on contact with your skin, leaving it silky smooth and not greasy.

Mango butter is a powerful and natural ingredient in body butter recipes and perfect for dry or sunburned skins. It moisturizes and nourishes the skin almost instantly and is frequently used with or as a substitute for cocoa and shea butter.

PREP TIME: 20 MINUTES

COOK TIME: 5 MINUTES

TOTAL TIME: 25 MINUTES

MAKES: 300 ML / 10 OZ

INGREDIENTS

- 12 tablespoons of organic unrefined mango butter
- 2 tablespoons of organic refined shea butter
- 6 tablespoons of organic safflower oil
- 1 teaspoon of arrowroot powder optional and to make it less greasy.
- 15 drops of roman chamomile essential oil
- 3 drops of bergamot Bergaptene free essential oil
- 10 drops of patchouli essential oil
- Glass Salve Containers– You can also find glass cream containers on amazon.com and amazon.ca

INSTRUCTIONS

- Put the shea and mango butter in a glass or metal bowl inside a pan filled with water on low heat so they starts melting slowly.
- Once melted add the safflower oil and mix well.
- Put the bowl the freezer for 5 to 10 minutes, depending on the temperature of your freezer. You want the mixture to not be completely frozen but thick enough so it is not liquid.
- If it's a soft paste then its ready to whip!
- Then take it out of the freezer and start whipping with an electric whip on low speed.
- Add the arrowroot powder if desired. This is optional but will help have a light feeling and texture on the skin.
- Make sure you wear an apron and that the bowl is deep enough so the butter does not start flying around everywhere in the kitchen!
- Begin whipping your mixture on low speed until it becomes fluffy.
- Once the mixture is fluffy, increase the speed to medium until it becomes whipped to the desired stage.
- Add essential oils if desired at the end and whip for 1 min or less.
- Your butter will have a very fluffy and light consistency, like a nice whipped cream!

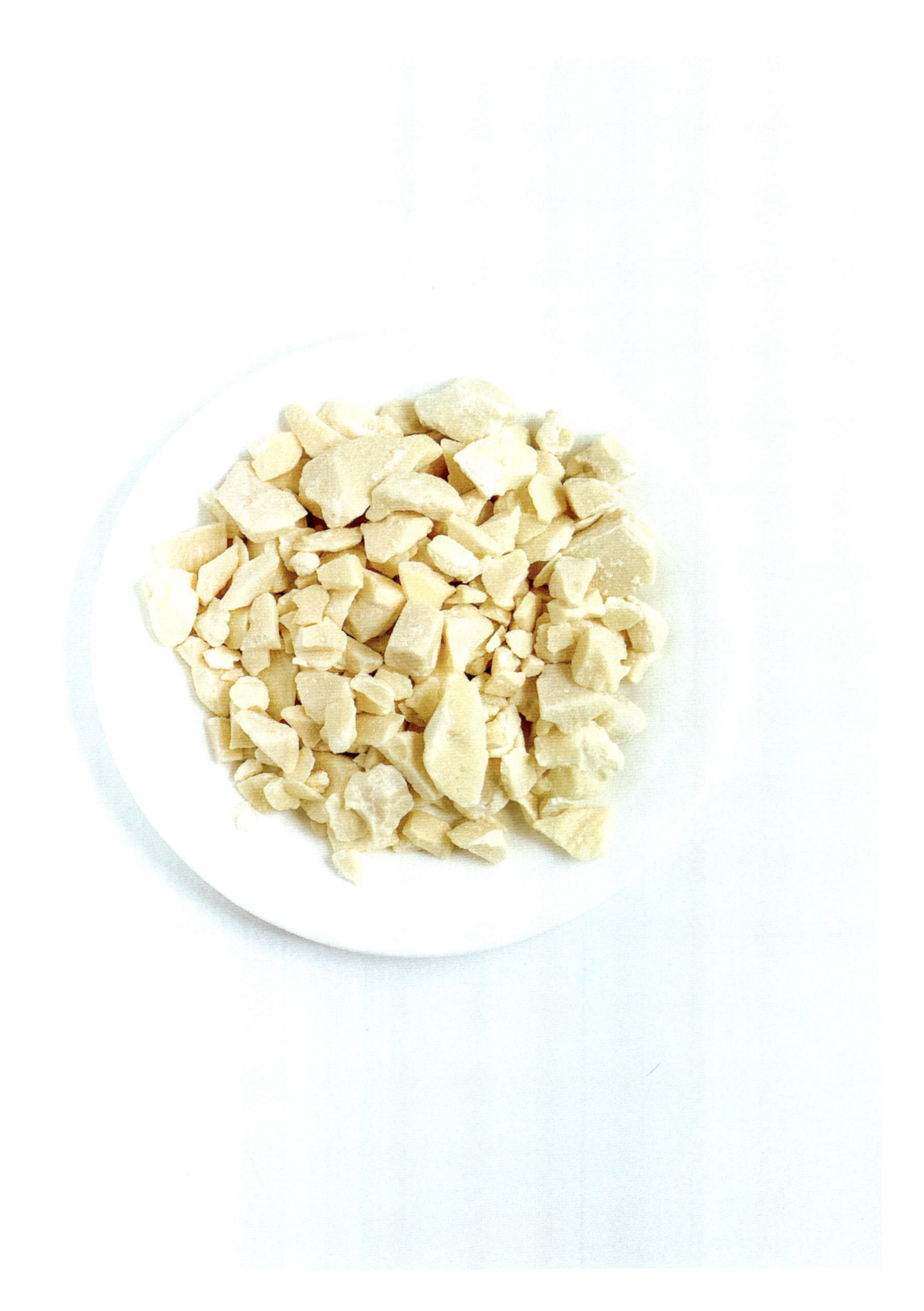

COCOA BODY BUTTER RECIPE

BODY BUTTER RECIPES

*T*his cocoa butter lotion recipe contains no beeswax and is easily done whipped. Cocoa Butter is naturally rich in Vitamin E as well as a number of other vitamins and minerals. Vitamin E helps to soothe, hydrate, and balance the skin and also provides the skin collagen which assists with wrinkles and other signs of aging. It is a rich body butter perfect for dry skin and for preventing stretch marks.

If you would like the chocolate scent, make sure you buy unrefined cocoa butter, the refined version will lose its yummy natural chocolate scent!

PREP TIME: 30 MINUTES

COOK TIME: 5 MINUTES

TOTAL TIME: 35 MINUTES

MAKES: 160 ML / 5.4 OZ

INGREDIENTS

- 4 tablespoons organic raw cocoa butter
- 6 tablespoons organic Camellia seed oil or safflower oil
- 1 tablespoon of organic pure aloe vera juice
- 16 drops of Grapeseed extract as a natural preservative (0.5%)
- ¼ teaspoon of raw natural silk protein powder (Optional)
- 10 drops of organic lavender oil

INSTRUCTIONS

- To make this cocoa butter lotion recipe, add the cocoa butter and camellia seed oil to your double boiler on low heat until they are melted.
- Once melted, take it off the heat, add the tablespoon of aloe vera and the silk protein (optional) and start whipping with an electric mixer for two minutes.
- Put the bowl into the freezer for 13 minutes. (You may need to adjust the time in the freezer depending on how cold your freezer is. If the butter is too hard to be mixed, just leave it a few minutes at room temperature.)
- Take the bowl out the freezer and start whipping with the electric mixer, you will see that it turns white and fluffy right away, continue whipping for 2-4 minutes. Be careful not to over whip or it will seize!
- Add the essential oils, grapeseed oil extract and whip again for a few seconds.
- Pour the cocoa body butter in a glass jar.

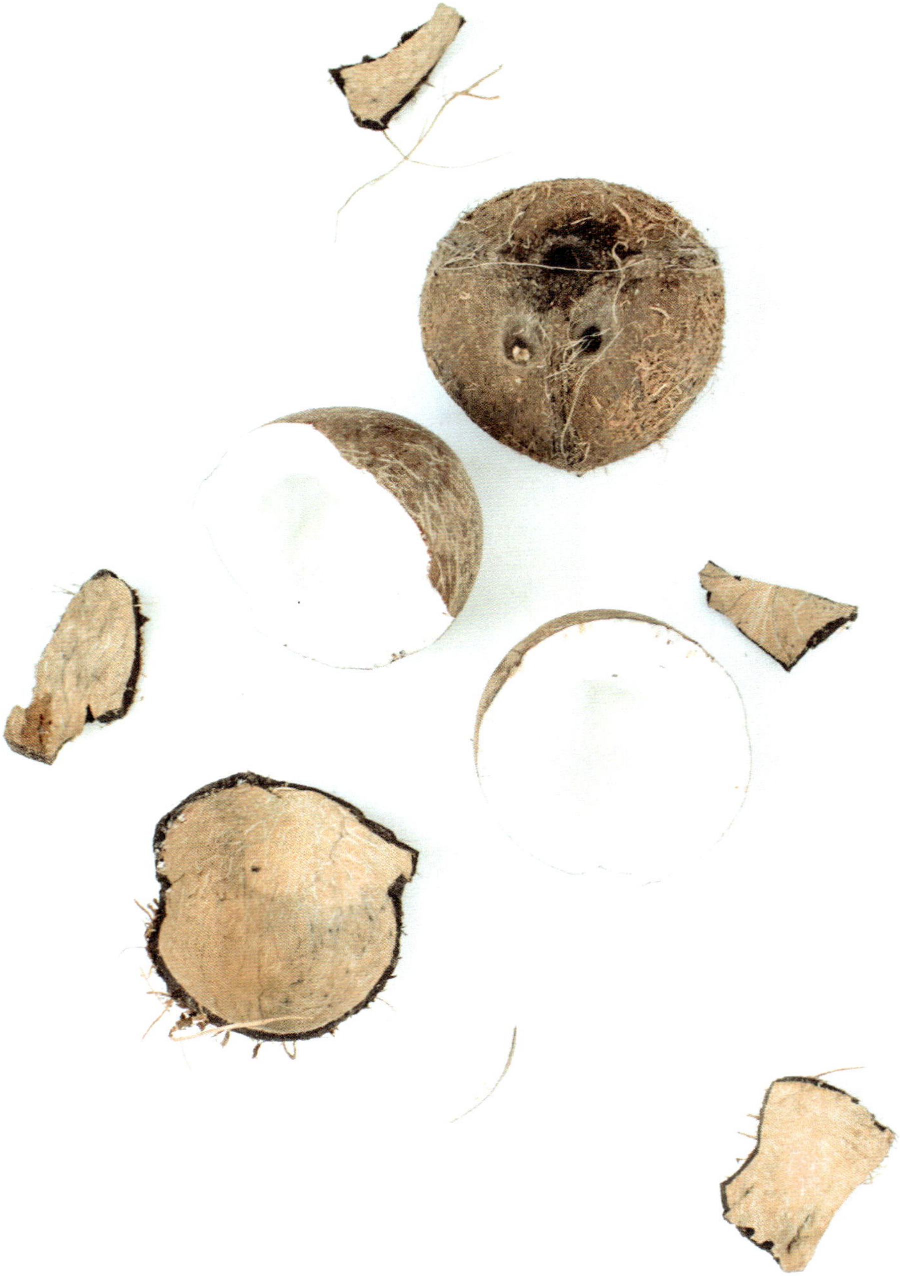

COCONUT BODY BUTTER

BODY BUTTER RECIPES

This is an easy coconut oil body butter recipe and you can whip it in max 20 minutes in your kitchen. It's a great body butter to fight against dry and flaky skin. Be sure to use unrefined coconut oil if you like the natural coconut scent. It also works well on dry and coarse hair to smooth freeze and moisturize. Just remember a little goes a long way!

PREP TIME: 15 MINUTES

COOK TIME: 5 MINUTES

TOTAL TIME: 20 MINUTES

MAKES: 160 ML / 5.4 OZ

INGREDIENTS

- 4 tablespoons of sunflower oil
- 2 tablespoons of refined shea butter
- 2 tablespoons of cocoa butter
- 3 tablespoons of coconut oil
- 0.5 teaspoon of carnauba wax
- 5 drops of palmarosa essential oil
- 5 drops of frankincense essential oil
- 3 drops of ylang ylang essential oil

INSTRUCTIONS

- Melt cocoa butter, coconut oil, shea butter and carnauba wax in a double boiler.
- Once melted, add the sunflower oil.
- Put the recipient in the freezer for 13-18 mins, until the ingredients have hardened but are not completely frozen.
- Take it out of the freezer and start mixing with a hand blender until it is nice and creamy.
- Add the essential oils if you wish.
- Pour into nice containers.
- Voila, you have made an all-natural and organic coconut oil body butter recipe!

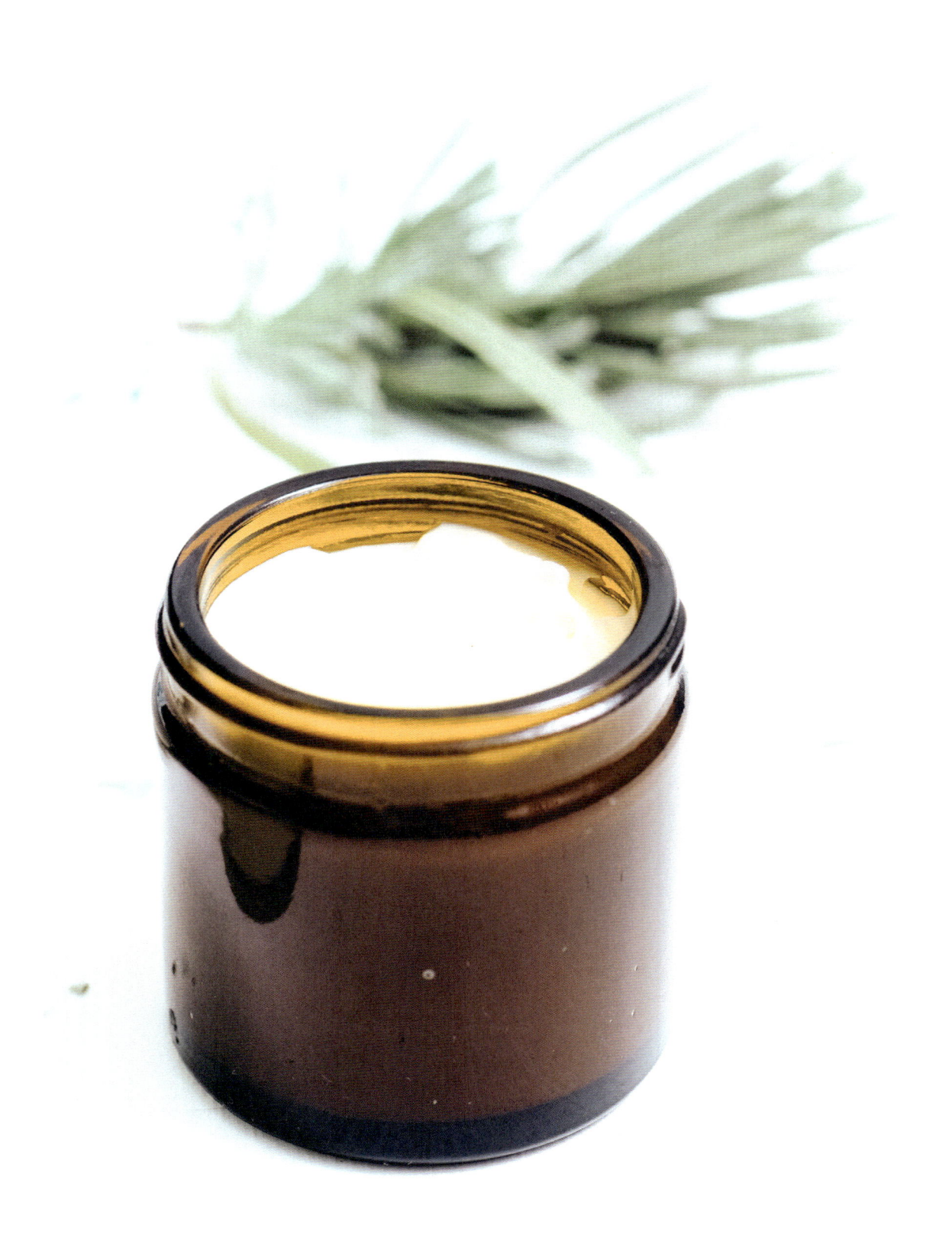

GALEN COLD CREAM

BODY CREAM RECIPES

The invention of cold cream is credited to Galen, a physician in the second century from Greece. This cold cream is thick and softens when it touches the skin. It is perfect for dry skin on elbow, feet, and knees and also perfect for natural ways of removing makeup and to avoid dry skin.

PREP TIME: 15 MINUTES

COOK TIME: 10 MINUTES

TOTAL TIME: 25 MINUTES

MAKES: 100ML OR 3 OZ

INGREDIENTS

- 9 teaspoons of rosewater
- 9 teaspoons of almond oil
- 2 teaspoons of beeswax
- 10 drops of grapeseed extract as a natural preservative (0.5%)
- 20 drops rose otto essential oils

INSTRUCTIONS

- Combine the oils in your double boiler (or in a stainless steel or glass recipient inside a pan filled with water) on low heat and wait until everything is melted.
- At the same time, put the water in another double boiler on low heat so that it reaches the same temperature as the oils.
- Once the oil and beeswax are melted, take it off the heat and start whipping with an electric mixer for a few minutes while adding the rosewater spoon by spoon.
- Make sure your mixer is set on low speed.
- You can also use a hand whip if you prefer but it is more work!
- After 2 to 5 minutes, the liquid will soon turn into a cream as you progressively add the water.
- Once you have reached the creamy consistency desired, add the grapeseed extract and essential oils and mix well.
- Scoop the cream in a sterile glass recipient and allow cooling at room temperature before putting the cap on.

Tip **BEESWAX IS HERE AN EFFECTIVE EMULSIFIER** that binds water and oil. The only trick is that you have to be careful with the ratio water vs oil. If you put too much water, your cream will separate!

ORGANIC BEAUTY RECIPES BY EVE

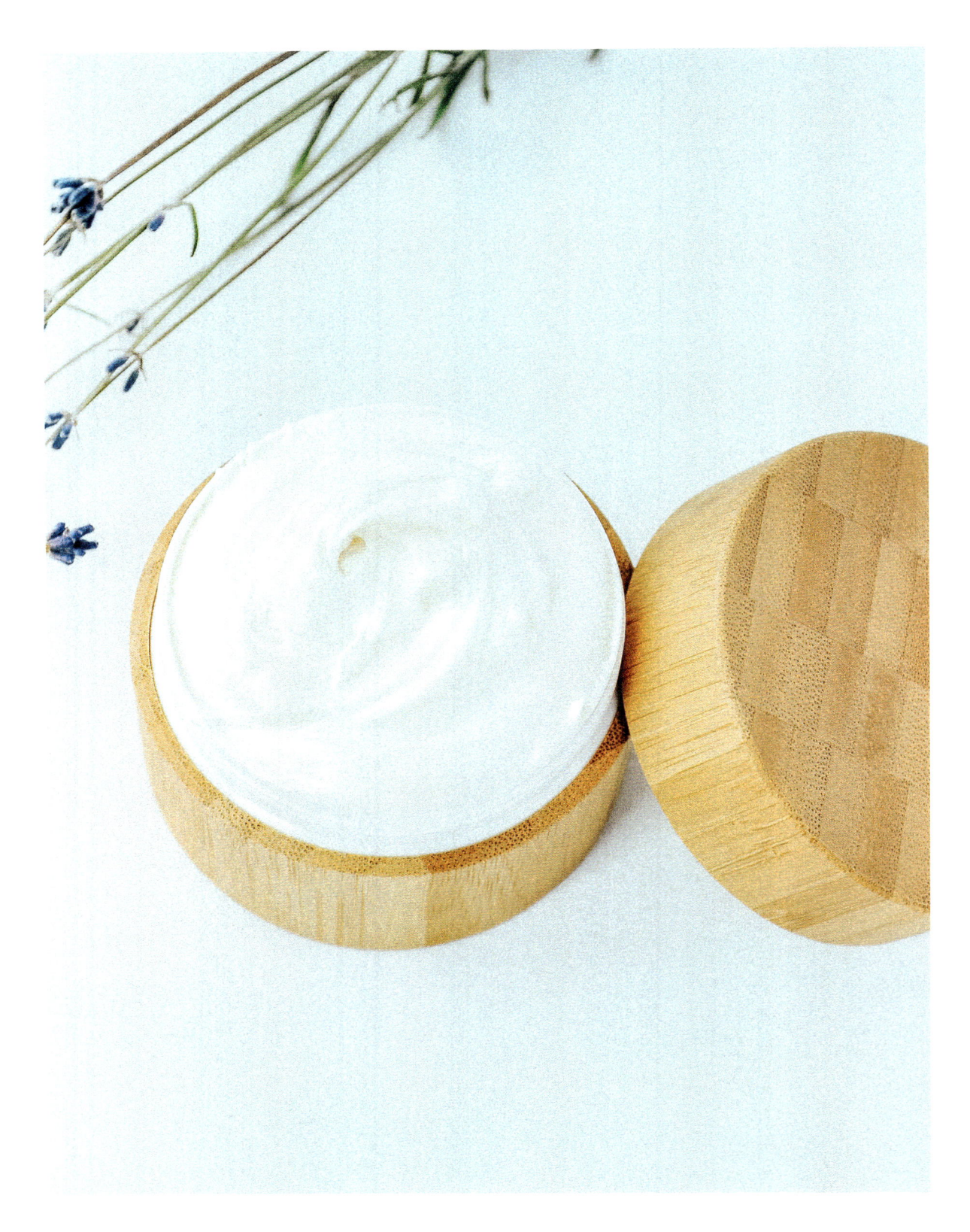

HOMEMADE BODY CREAM

BODY CREAM RECIPES

My homemade moisturizer tutorial is easy to follow with only four ingredients, apricot kernel oil, beeswax, rosewater (hydrosol) and cocoa butter. By picking high-power moisturizing oil and butter that provide plenty of nourishment, it delivers glowing skin and maximum hydration. This body cream is perfect if you have dry skin and need extra nourishment.

The texture is fondant, melts on the touch and is easy to apply. Plus it absorbs very well into the skin and does not leave a greasy feeling. You don't need a lot of this DIY natural cream to moisturize your skin!

PREP TIME: 30 MINUTES

COOK TIME: 10 MINUTES

TOTAL TIME: 40 MINUTES

MAKES: 230 ML / 7.7 OZ

INGREDIENTS

- 1 tablespoon of organic rose water
- 4 tablespoons of organic cocoa butter
- 10 tablespoons of organic apricot kernel oil
- 1 tablespoon of organic beeswax pellets
- 23 drops of grapeseed extract as a natural preservative (0.5%)
- 10 drops of lavender essential oil (optional)

INSTRUCTIONS

- Combine all the oils, cocoa butter & beeswax to your double boiler (basically put an aluminum bowl or pyrex in a pan filled with water) on low heat until they are melted.
- Add the rose water, mix well.
- Once all the ingredients are melted, take your bowl out of the heat and put it in another recipient bowl filled with cold water, ideally with ice to speed up the emulsification process.
- Start mixing with an electric hand blender like this one until you get a liquid cream consistency.
- To whip this butter and make it fondant, put the bowl in the freezer for 10 minutes.
- Then, use the hand blender to mix the cream again.
- Add the essential oil if desired.
- Pour in a glass jar container.

72   ORGANIC BEAUTY RECIPES BY EVE

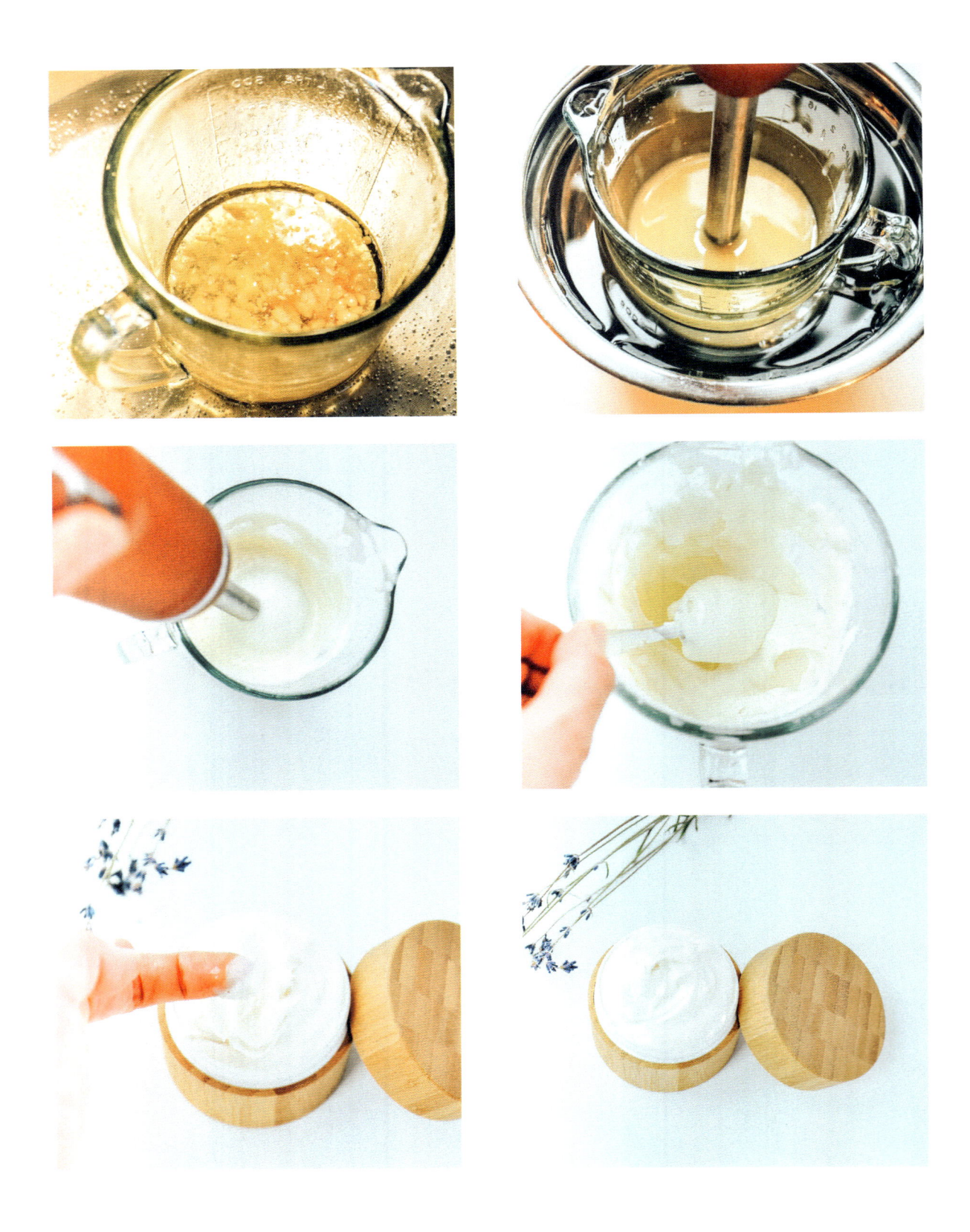

HOMEMADE BODY CREAM TUTORIAL STEP BY STEP

Step 1

Combine all the oils, cocoa butter & beeswax to your double boiler on low heat until they are melted.

Add the rose water, mix well.

Step 2

Once all the ingredients are melted, take your bowl out of the heat and put it in another recipient bowl filled with cold water, ideally with ice to speed up the emulsification process.

Start mixing with an electric hand blender like this one until you get a liquid cream consistency.

Step 3

To whip this butter and make it fondant, put the bowl in the freezer for 10 minutes.

Then, use the hand blender to mix the cream again.

Add the essential oil if desired. it does help with preservation time.

Step 4

Add the grapeseed oil extract and essential oil.

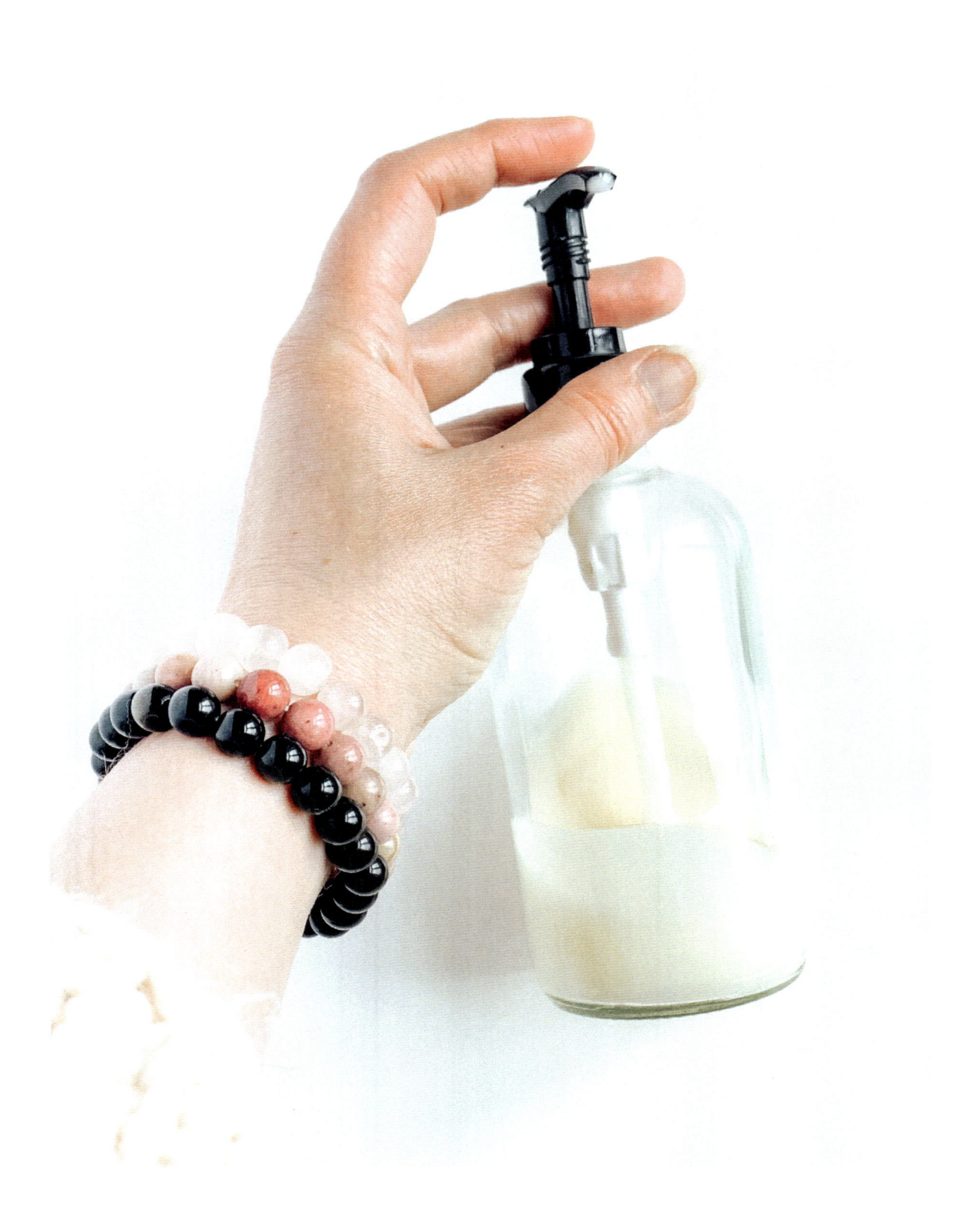

HAND LOTION FOR DRY HANDS (PUMPABLE!)

BODY CREAM RECIPES

*If you are struggling with the damage that winter has done on your hands, then I have the perfect DIY beauty product to make: my homemade hand lotion. You can learn how to make your own hand moisturizer with only 4 ingredients, beeswax, almond oil, rosewater and shea butter.

The high concentration of fatty acids of shea butter coupled with a high dose of vitamins in it is what makes it such an amazing moisturizer.

This hand lotion is also pumpable!

PREP TIME: 10 MINUTES

COOK TIME: 10 MINUTES

TOTAL TIME: 20 MINUTES

MAKES: 140 ML / 4.7 OZ

INGREDIENTS

- 1 teaspoon of beeswax pellets
- 16 teaspoons of sweet almond oil
- 1 teaspoon of refined shea butter
- 10 teaspoons rose hydrosol
- 1 teaspoon of vegetable glycerin
- 15 drops Grapefruit seed extract as a natural preservative.
- 20 drops lavender essential oil optional

INSTRUCTIONS

- Combine all the oil, shea butter & beeswax to your double boiler on low to medium heat until they are melted.
- Add the hydrosol. Mix well and ensure all ingredients are melted and in liquid form.
- Take your double boiler out of the heat and place in another recipient filled with cold water. No need for ice. Make sure the water does not get inside your double boiler where the ingredients are.
- Start whipping with a hand whip until you get the creamy consistency desired. It should take 2 to 5 minutes max. Once the emulsion has appeared and your ingredients turned into a liquid cream, you are done. Make sure you can see traces of the whip in the cream when you turn it around.
- Add the essential oils, the glycerin and the grapefruit seed extract and mix well.
- Pour immediately in a glass jar container such as a pumpable lotion container.

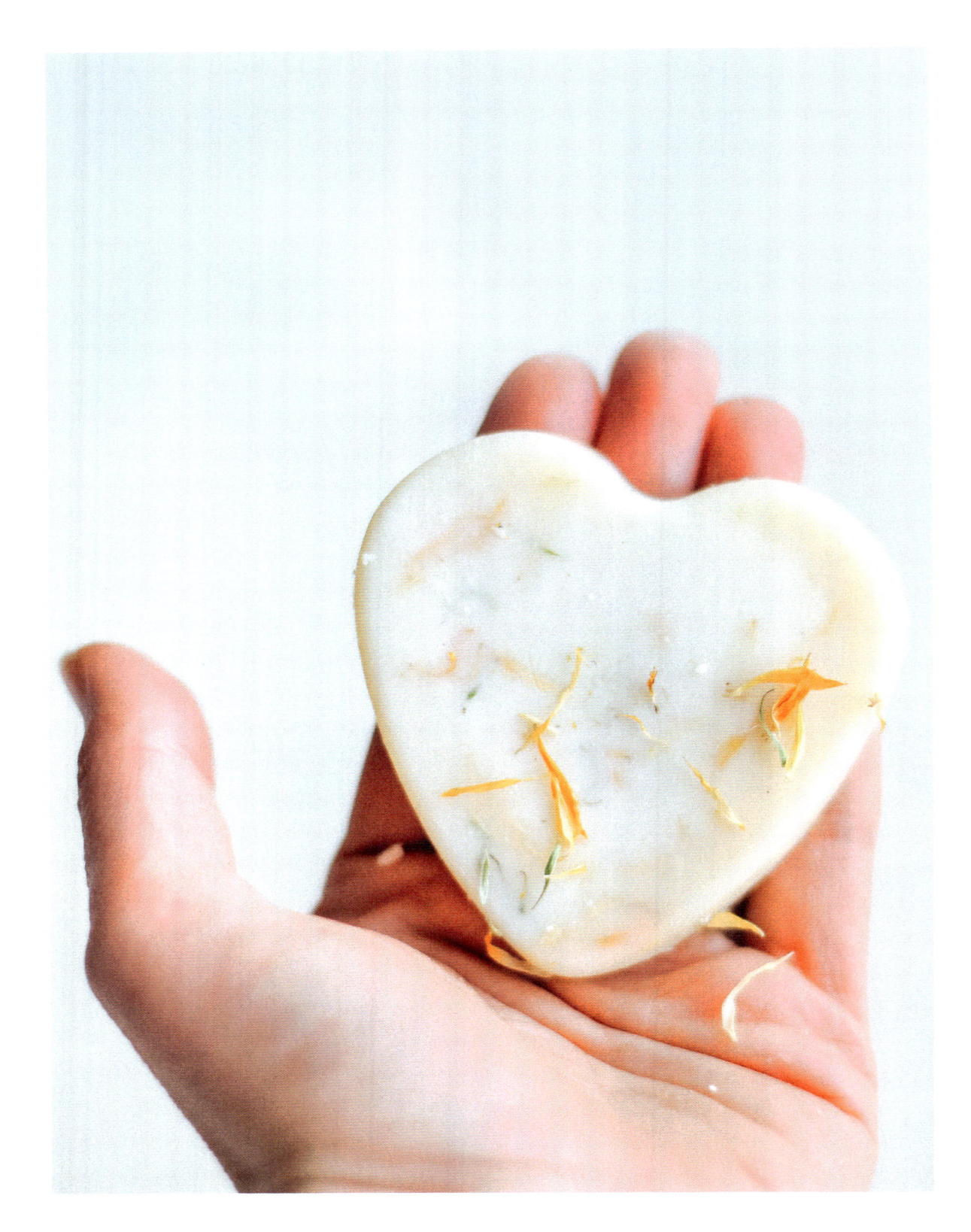

HOW TO MAKE LOTION BARS WITOUT BEESWAX

LOTION AND MASSAGE BARS RECIPES

This homemade lotion bar is super silky and buttery. The texture is light, smooth and feels like a luxurious massage on the skin. I will teach you how to make lotion bars without beeswax. It's vegan and is also great for stretch marks!

PREP TIME: 10 MINUTES

COOK TIME: 5 MINUTES

TOTAL TIME: 15 MINUTES

MAKES: 2 OZ / 60 ML OR 2 LOTION BARS

INGREDIENTS

- 2 tablespoons of organic cocoa butter
- 1 tablespoon pure refined organic shea butter
- 1 teaspoon of organic safflower oil
- 1 tablespoon of dried lavender buds or dried calendula flowers (optional)
- 5 drops of lavender essential oil
- 5 drops of frankincense essential oil
- 5 drops of rose geranium essential oil
- Heart shape silicon mold

INSTRUCTIONS

- Melt butter and oil in a double boiler
- One melted take it off the heat and mix well.
- Add dried lavender flower or dried calendula flower if desired.
- Add the essential oils if you wish. Take care of not adding the essential oil too soon as they are volatile and can evaporate if your ingredients are too warm.
- Pour in a silicon or soap mold right away.
- Put in the fridge for 1 hour until it has completely solidified.

How to use your lotion bar

- Rub all over your skin. It will melt on body contact.
- You can leave these homemade beauty bars at room temperature. They are made to stay hard but you should keep in a cool, dry place out of direct sunlight.
- This will make two solid lotion bars.

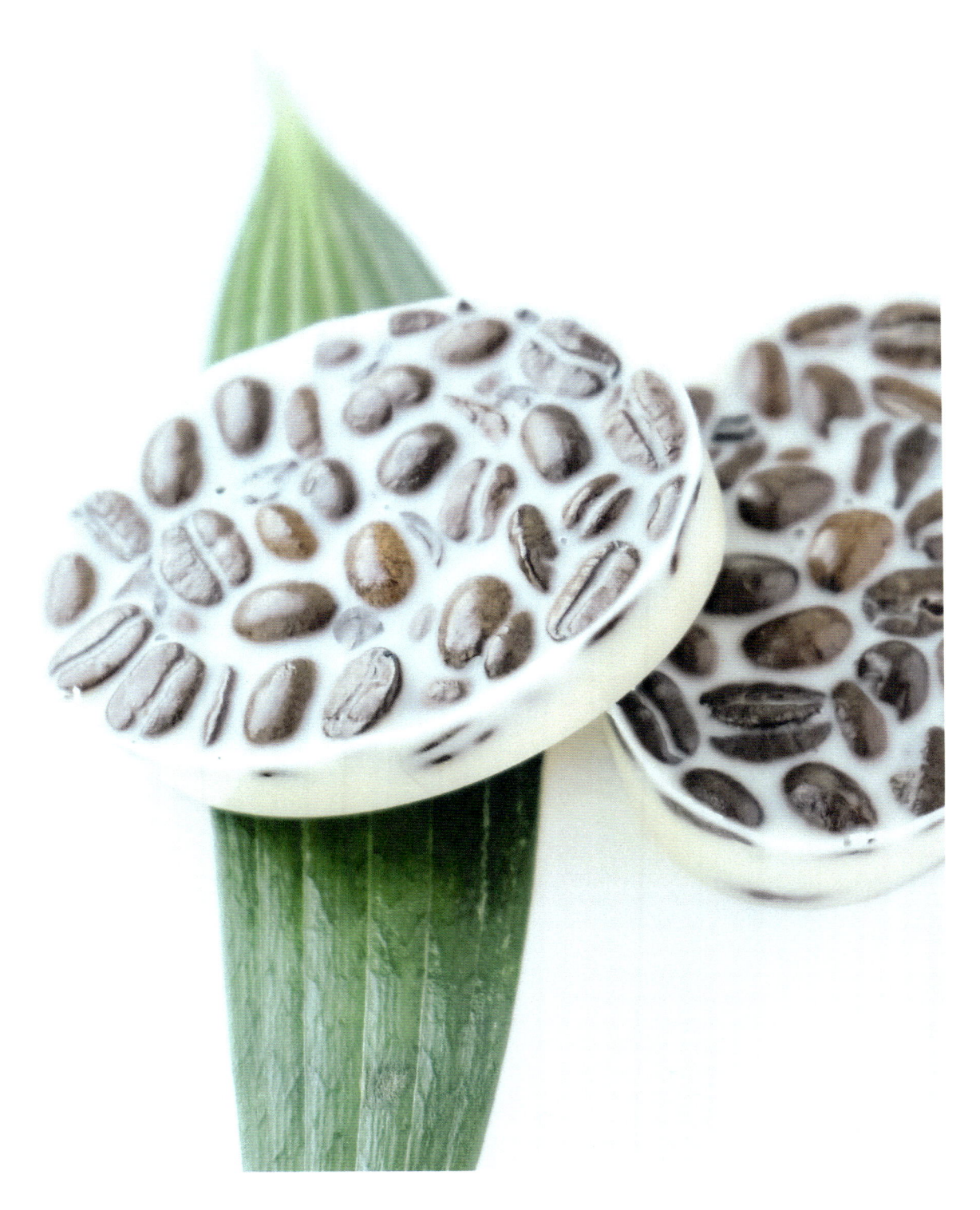

DIY COFFEE MASSAGE BAR AGAINST CELLULITE

LOTION AND MASSAGE BARS RECIPES

I've created this recipe with moisturizing mango and cocoa butters, coffee beans and uplifting essential oils such as grapefruit that will melt straight into your skin, leaving you feeling alert, rejuvenated and stress-free. The coffee beans will help to massage your skin gently and get your lymphatic system moving. The combined scent of coffee and grapefruit essential oil has an acidic and citrusy smell that will leave you wanting for more, it is quite addicting!

PREP TIME: 10 MINUTES

COOK TIME: 5 MINUTES

TOTAL TIME: 15 MINUTES

MAKES: 3 OZ / 88 ML OR 2 LOTION BARS

INGREDIENTS

- 1 tablespoon organic mango butter
- 1 tablespoon of organic cocoa butter
- 1 tablespoon of coconut oil
- 3 tablespoons of natural beeswax
- 10 drops grapefruit essential oil
- 5 drops Juniper Berry essential oil
- 5 drops geranium essential oil
- 1 tablespoon of whole coffee beans or enough to fill the bottom of the mold

INSTRUCTIONS

- Melt butter, oil, and beeswax in a double boiler on low heat.
- Add the coffee beans in the bottom of your silicone mold so it covers the entire bottom part.
- Once the beeswax and butter are melted, remove from the heat and add the essential oils, mix well.
- Pour right away in your favorite soap mold.
- Put in the fridge for 1 hour.
- Un-mold and it's ready to use!

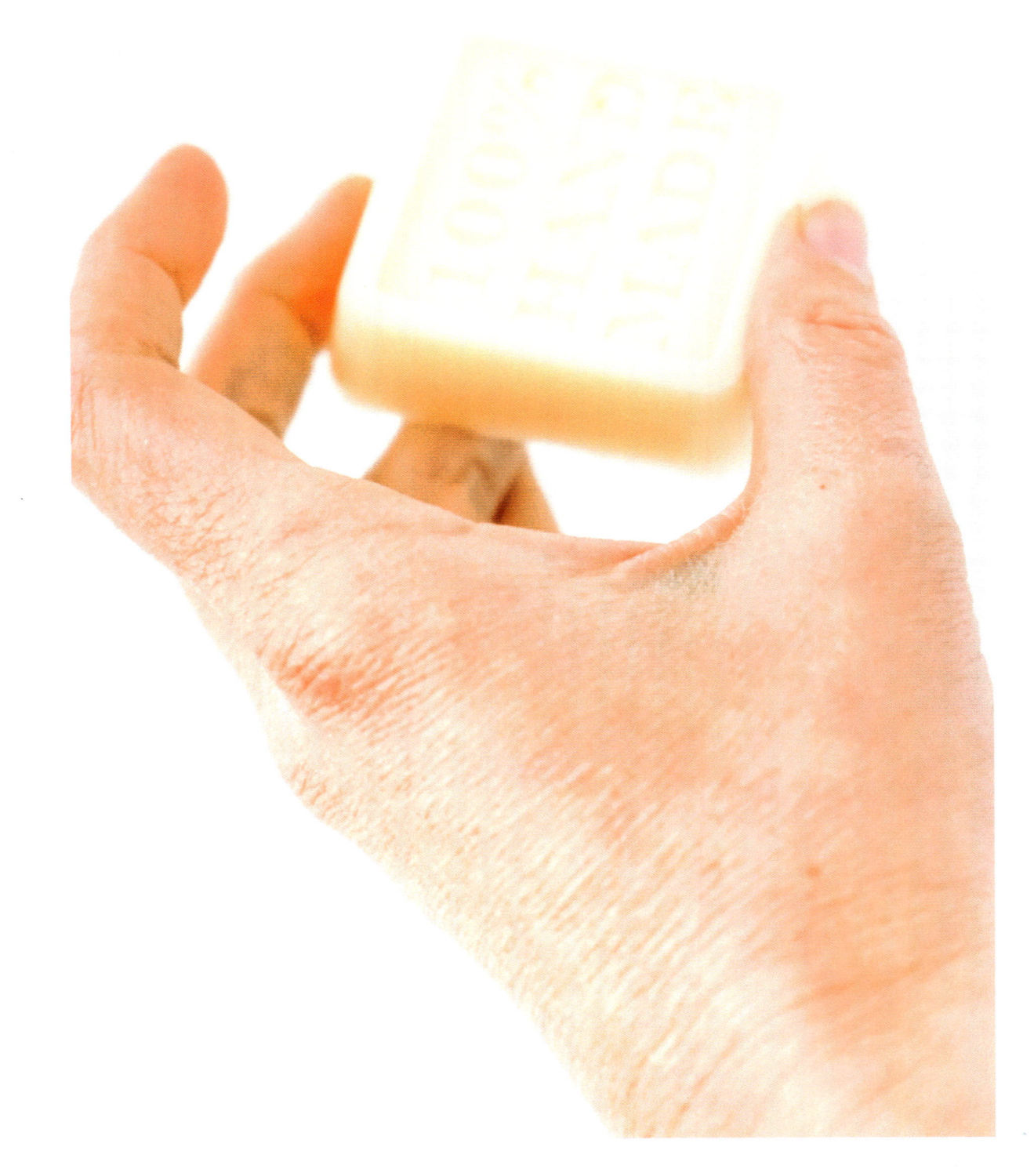

HOMEMADE LOTION BAR FOR DRY SKIN

LOTION AND MASSAGE BARS RECIPES

My lotion bar for dry skin has only 3 ingredients, coconut oil, beeswax, and raw shea butter. It's important to use the organic and raw (unrefined) version for each ingredient to have the highest quality possible. These homemade lotion bars are very easy to make, you can't mess it up, simply melt and pour!

PREP TIME: 10 MINUTES

COOK TIME: 10 MINUTES

TOTAL TIME: 20 MINUTES

MAKES: 2 OZ / 60 ML OR 2 LOTION BARS

INGREDIENTS

- 2 tablespoons of organic raw Shea butter
- 1 tablespoon of organic beeswax pellets
- 1 tablespoon of organic coconut oil
- 1 handmade soap mold

INSTRUCTIONS

- Melt butter, oil, and beeswax in a double boiler on low heat.
- Once melted, pour right away in your favorite soap mold.
- Put in the fridge for 1 hour.
- Un-mold and it's ready to use!

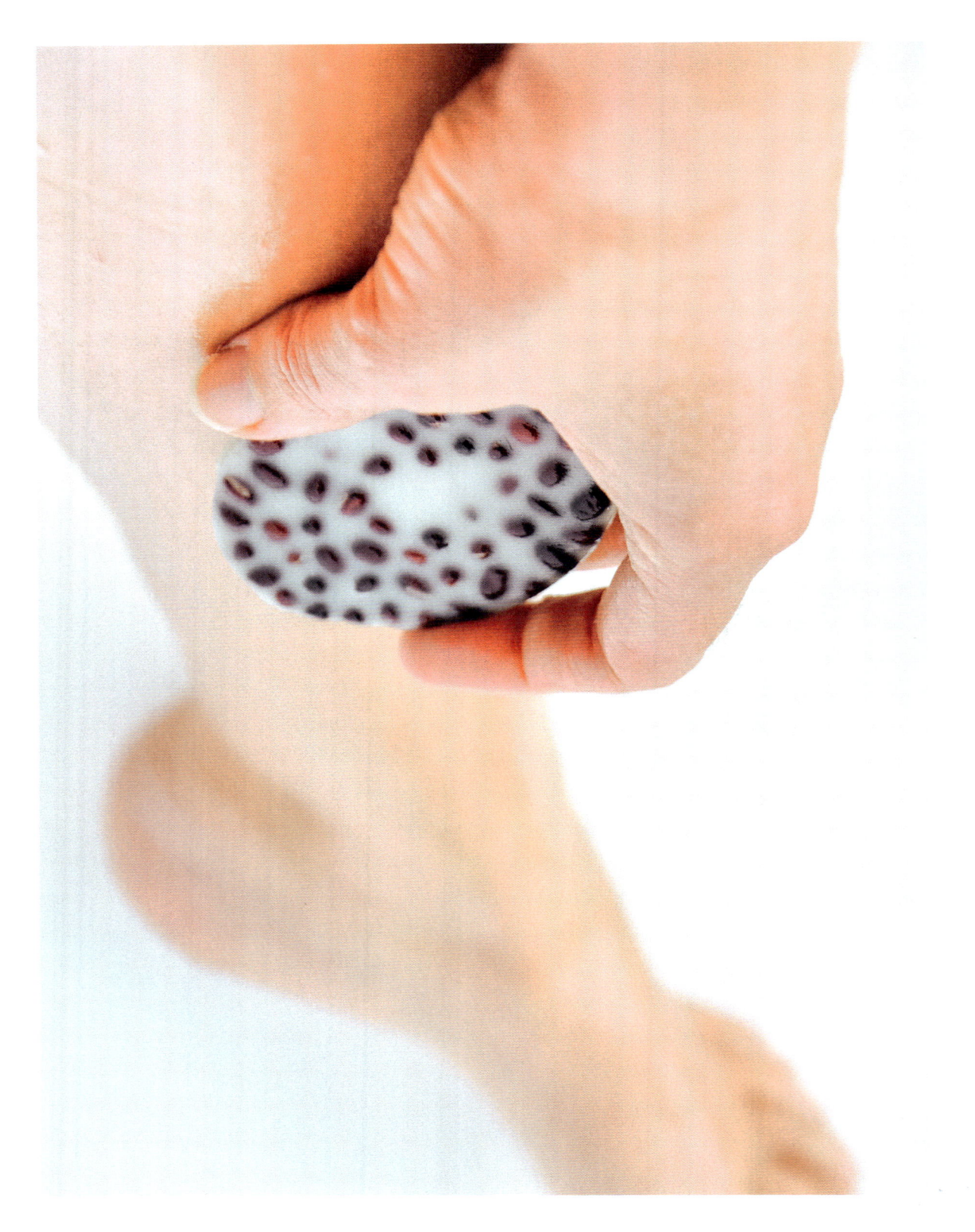

DIY MASSAGE BAR FOR SORE MUSLES

LOTION AND MASSAGE BARS RECIPES

This DIY massage bar for sore muscles is similar to popular brand name product, but without the synthetic fragrance and other additives. I've used dried aduki beans, shea butter, cocoa butter, jojoba oil, coconut oil and beeswax.

There is also peppermint essential oil and cinnamon leaf essential oil for their soothing and cooling/warming properties for sore muscles.

PREP TIME: 10 MINUTES

COOK TIME: 10 MINUTES

TOTAL TIME: 20 MINUTES

MAKES: 2 OZ / 60 ML OR 2 LOTION BARS

INGREDIENTS

- 1 tablespoon organic refined Shea butter
- 1 tablespoon of organic cocoa butter
- 1 teaspoon of jojoba oil
- 2 teaspoons of coconut oil
- 1 tablespoon of natural beeswax
- 10 drops peppermint essential oil
- 5 drops cinnamon leaf essential oil
- 5 drops lavender essential oil
- 1 tablespoon of whole adzuki beans or enough to fill the bottom of the mold

INSTRUCTIONS

- Melt butter, oil, and beeswax in a double boiler on low heat.
- Add the adzuki beans in the bottom of your mold so it covers the entire bottom part.
- Once the beeswax and butter are melted, add the essential oils, mix well.
- Pour right away in your favorite soap mold.
- Put in the fridge for 1 hour.
- Un-mold and it's ready to use!

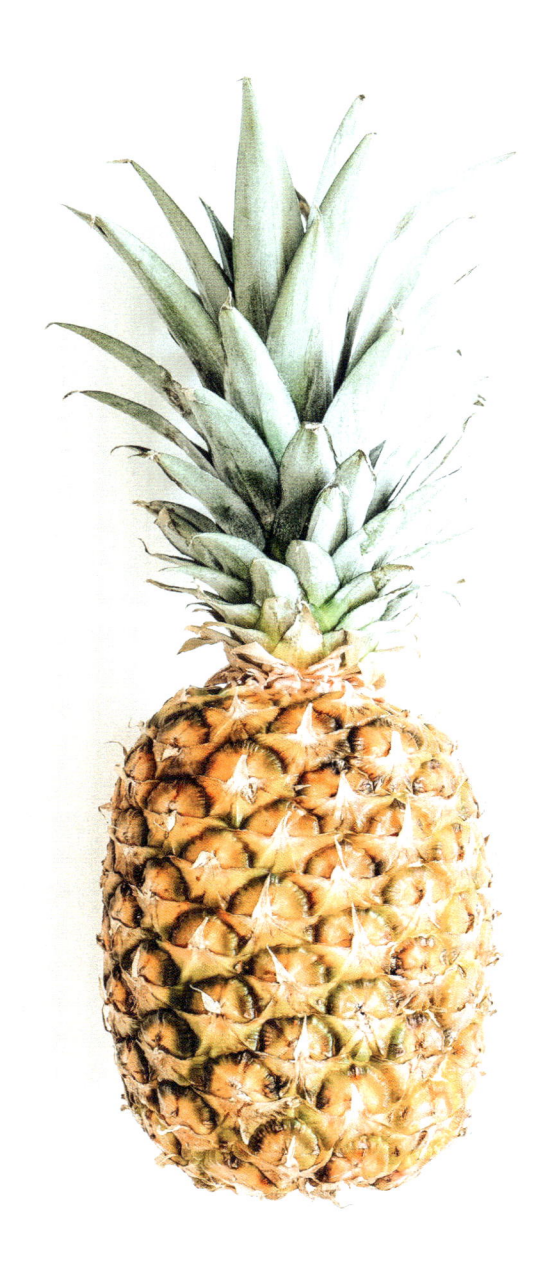

COCONUT AND PINEAPLE BODY SCRUB

BODY SCRUB RECIPES

*T*his body scrub has simple ingredients and includes pineapple which is wonderful for the skin; it contains alpha-hydroxyl acids and is full of vitamins (a, b1, b6, C). The enzyme bromelain in the pineapple has anti-inflammatory properties, will polish dead cells, regenerate your skin and buff it! Coconut butter is great for skin hydration and the polenta or corn meal is a cheap ingredient perfect for exfoliation.

This is a scrub that needs be done fresh and used the day of. Enjoy your spa day at home!

PREP TIME: 5 MINUTES

TOTAL TIME: 5 MINUTES

MAKES: 1 APPLICATION

INGREDIENTS

- 1 cup of Pineapple Blended
- 1 cup polenta or cornmeal
- 1 cup of dry coconut meat shredded
- 2 teaspoons organic cold pressed coconut butter

INSTRUCTIONS

- Blend the pineapple in a fast blender to puree it (make sure you have removed the skin of course!).
- Add the Polenta and the shredded coconut and the coconut butter.
- Blend well.
- Apply and massage the body scrub everywhere on your body (avoiding sensitive parts) while in your bathtub so you don't make a mess.
- If possible leave it on skin for 5 to 10 minutes then rinse!

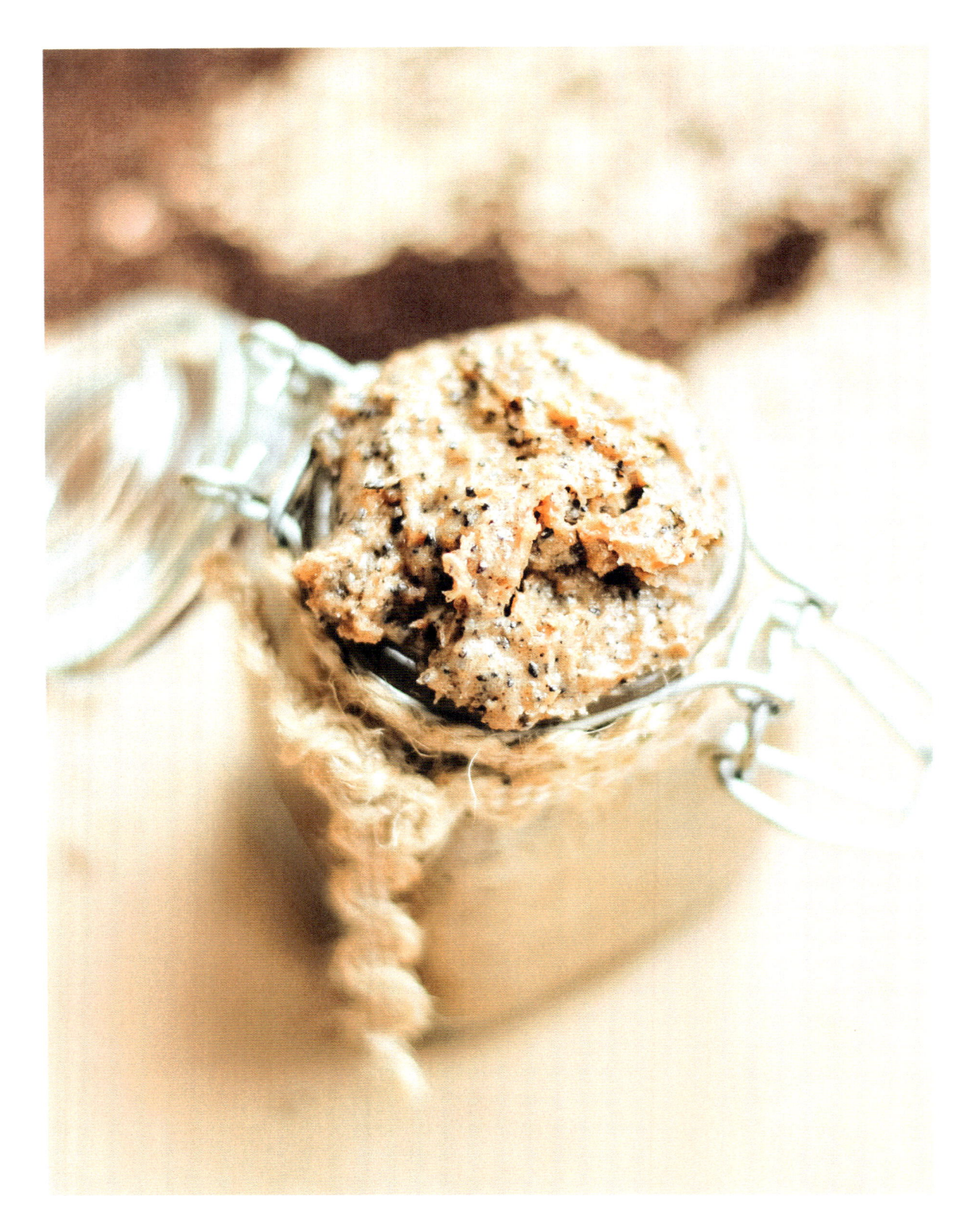

COFFEE BODY SCRUB

BODY SCRUB RECIPES

Oh coffee... While I don't drink it, the smell always leaves me wanting for more! This coffee body scrub recipe will leave yours skin smooth and well hydrated. Coffee basically "buffs" your skin and gives it a nice golden glow. Plus it can reduce the appearance of cellulite!

Bottom line, this coffee body scrub smells amazing and it's super easy and fun to make.

PREP TIME: 5 MINUTES

TOTAL TIME: 5 MINUTES

MAKES: 4 APPLICATIONS

INGREDIENTS

- 1/3 cup of organic whole brown sugar
- 1/3 cup organic coconut oil it needs to be cold and in solid form. If the coconut oil is melted put it in the fridge until it hardens.
- 1/3 cup of organic liquid castile soap like Dr Bronners
- 2 tablespoons of organic ground coffee

INSTRUCTIONS

- In a fast blender mix sugar and coconut oil until they are just blended for a few seconds. Don't mix too long as this will break down the sugar and melt the coconut oil.
- Pour the sugar and coconut oil in an aluminum bowl placed in a another bowl filled with cold iced water.
- Start whipping the scrub with an electric mixer until the scrub is fluffy and creamy
- Add the ground coffee and liquid soap until they are just combined.
- Put the scrub in a pretty container and use within 1 month.
- If it's hot (more than 25C) in your apartment, keep it in the fridge. Otherwise you can leave it at room temperature.
- Use weekly in the morning shower as body scrub, gently scrub your body but avoid sensitive areas.

Tip **THE COCONUT OIL IS A NATURAL WONDER TO HYDRATE YOUR SKIN BUT IS NOT SUCH A WONDER FOR YOUR BATH TUB.** Meaning, it will leave it greasy...! To flush the coconut oil from your bathtub, use hot water and wash it with your natural spray cleaner. Just make sure you don't run cold water as this will harden the coconut and might clog your pipes temporarily.

WORD OF CAUTION
If you have never used coffee on your skin before, it's always best to do a patch test in case you have an allergic reaction. Better be safe than sorry!

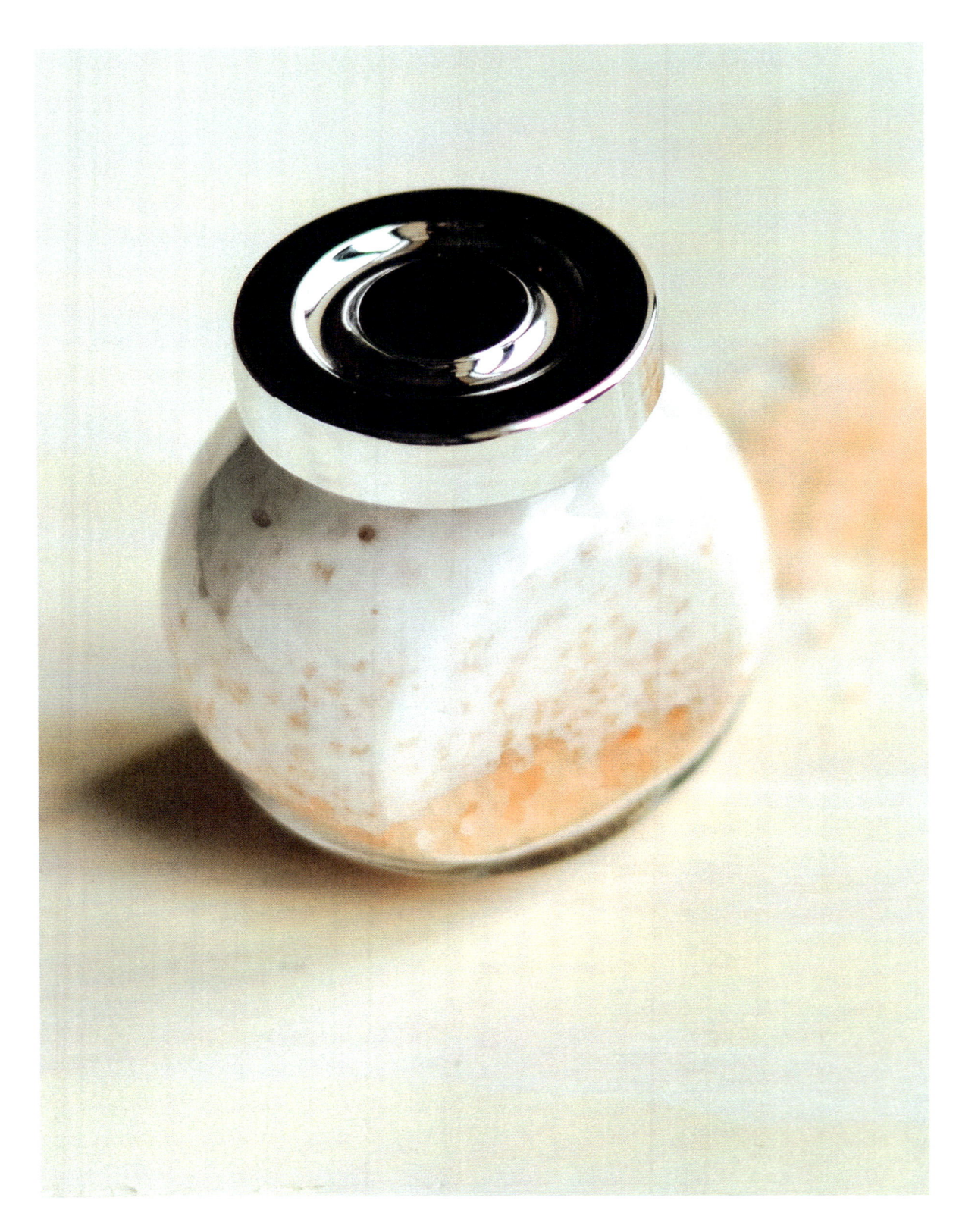

HYMALAYAN SEA SALT FOOD SCRUB & SOAK

BODY SCRUB RECIPES

I created this Himalayan Pink Salt DIY Foot Scrub & Soak Recipe to remove all those nasty dead and hard skins and so you can have baby smooth feet…

Himalayan Pink Salt has a rich mineral content that includes over 84 minerals including calcium, magnesium, potassium, copper and iron… This salt has a beautiful pink colour and is well known for its therapeutic properties, it will do wonders for your feet!

PREP TIME: 5 MINUTES

TOTAL TIME: 5 MINUTES

MAKES: 7.5 OZ / 221 ML

INGREDIENTS

- 5 tablespoons of pink Himalayan sea salt
- 10 tablespoons of organic coconut oil
- 1 teaspoon of baking soda with no aluminium please!
- 10 drops of organic grapefruit essential oil
- 10 drops of organic peppermint essential oil
- 10 drops of sweet orange essential oil

INSTRUCTIONS

- Whip the coconut oil with an electric hand whipper for a few minutes until it is white and fluffy.
- Ensure it is cold enough to be in solid form otherwise you won't be able to whip it. Put it in the fridge for 1 hour if needed.
- Combine the all the ingredients together and blend well.
- Then pour in a pretty glass container.
- Use a loofa or a glove to gently massage your feet for a few minutes with the scrub.
- Once you have scrubbed your feet, put them in warm water and add the rest of the DIY foot scrub if there are any left.
- Soak your feet for 15 minutes. Read a good book and relax!
- Scrub your feet for a few minutes again to remove the dead skins and then rinse well with water.

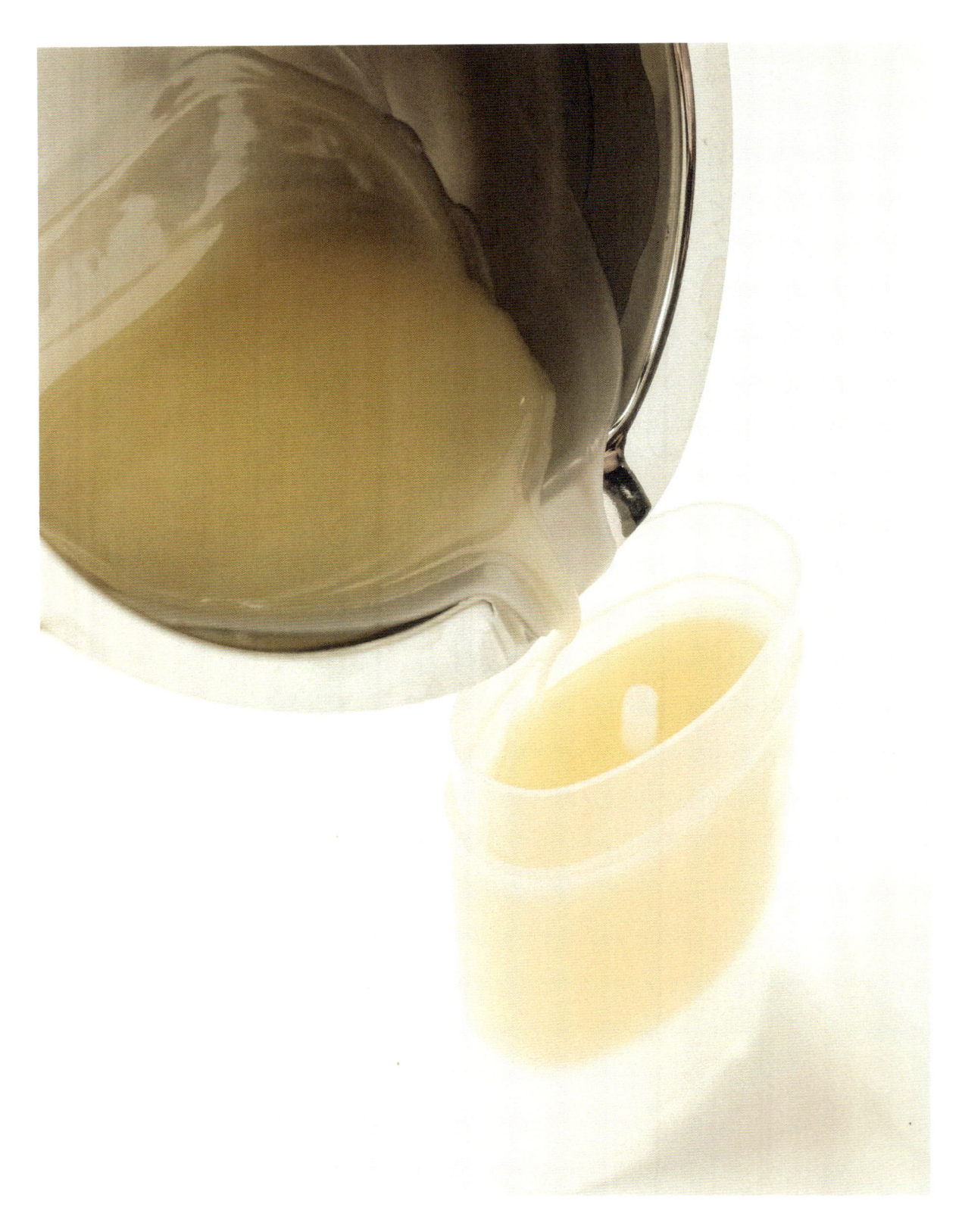

HOMEMADE DEODORANT WITHOUT BAKING SODA

DEODORANT RECIPE

*I*nstead of relying on baking soda, which often causes skin irritation, my homemade deodorant recipe focuses on nourishing oils like shea butter, gentle drying powders like arrowroot, and a blend of essential oils for an effective formula that will keep bacteria at bay and keep your armpit nice smelling!

PREP TIME: 10 MINUTES

COOK TIME: 10 MINUTES

TOTAL TIME: 20 MINUTES

MAKES: 2.5OZ / 75 ML

INGREDIENTS

- 2 tablespoons of Shea butter
- 3 tablespoons of Coconut oil
- 3 tablespoons of Beeswax pellets
- 1 tablespoon of Arrowroot powder
- 10 drops Lavender essential oil
- 10 drops Frankincense essential oil
- 10 drops rose geranium essential oil
- 10 drops Rosewood essential oil
- 1 empty deodorant stick

INSTRUCTIONS

- Melt beeswax, oils, and butter in a double boiler on low heat. If you do not have a double boiler, simply use an aluminum bowl placed in a pan filled with warm water.
- Add the arrowroot powder, mix well.
- Once melted, remove from heat, add the essential oils.
- Mix well.
- Pour immediately into the deodorant containers.
- Put it in the fridge for 2 hours until it has completely solidified.
- Apply on your clean armpit after your shower on dry skin.
- The shelf life of this deodorant is about 1 year, depending on the shelf life of the oils and you have used. It does not need to be refrigerated.

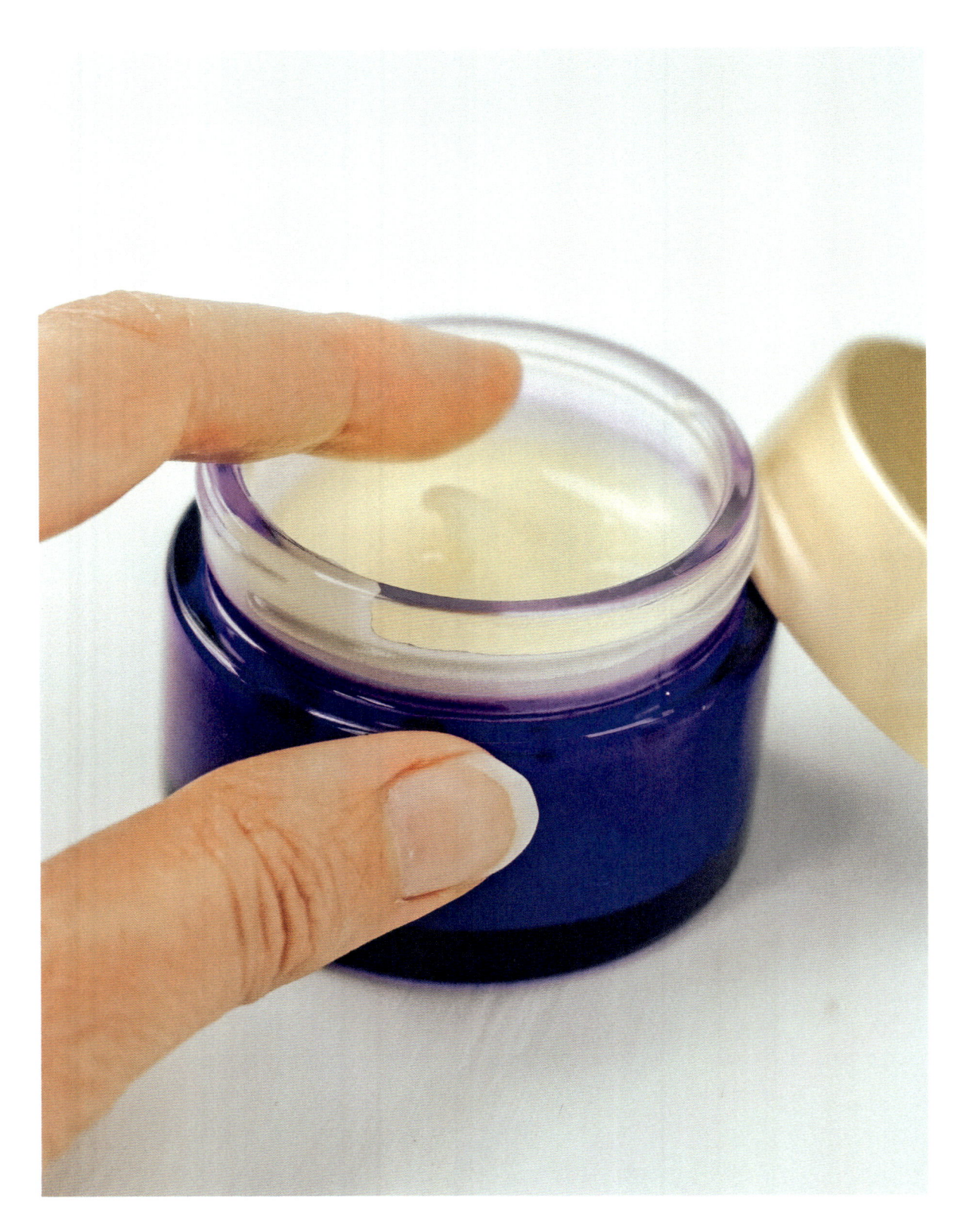

HOMEMADE SUNSCREEN WITHOUT TITANIUM DIOXIDE

SUNSCREEN RECIPE

With so many sunscreen products on the market filled with toxic ingredients, I wanted to make a great quality natural homemade sunscreen alternative using all organic products. The ingredients I used are pure cold-pressed jojoba oil, 100% organic red raspberry seed oil and raw shea butter that all have natural SPF. Since Jojoba and Red raspberry oil are a little on the pricey side, I recommend using this shea butter sunscreen only on your face. This DIY sunscreen is without zinc oxide and without titanium dioxide.

Also, my DIY sunscreen recipe does not contain beeswax so it is a vegan sunscreen and it can be done under 15 minutes!

Raspberry seed oil

Filled with hydrating properties to restore fine lines and improved parched skin, raspberry seed oil offers SPF ranging from 28-50 depending on the natural source. It's known to contain enough antioxidants to protect against UVA & UVB rays similar to Titanium Dioxide that's included in many mineral-based sunscreens.

PREP TIME: 10 MINUTES

TOTAL TIME: 10 MINUTES

MAKES: 7 OZ / 200 ML

INGREDIENTS

- 4 tablespoons organic shea butter
- 5 tablespoons raspberry seed oil
- 5 tablespoons jojoba oil
- Glass Salve Containers

INSTRUCTIONS

- Combine shea butter, raspberry seed oil and jojoba oil in a glass bowl.
- Start mixing the shea butter and oils with a hand immersion mixer to make the homemade sunscreen.
- Continue mixing until smooth, should take no more than 2 minutes to turn onto a cream.
- Pour into a pretty glass jar container.
- Use within 6 months and apply this homemade sunscreen on your face before going under the sun.
- Please note this is not a waterproof sunscreen!

Tip **USE COMMON SENSE UNDER THE SUN.** As much as we love staying out all morning under the beautiful sun, limiting direct sun exposure will help prevent any long-term sun damage. Reapply your homemade sunscreen every 30 minutes or so and always after you have been in the water. Cover up and shade your skin using a large hat, sunglasses, umbrella and loose clothing. Avoid sun tanning between 10am and 3pm when the sun is at its strongest!

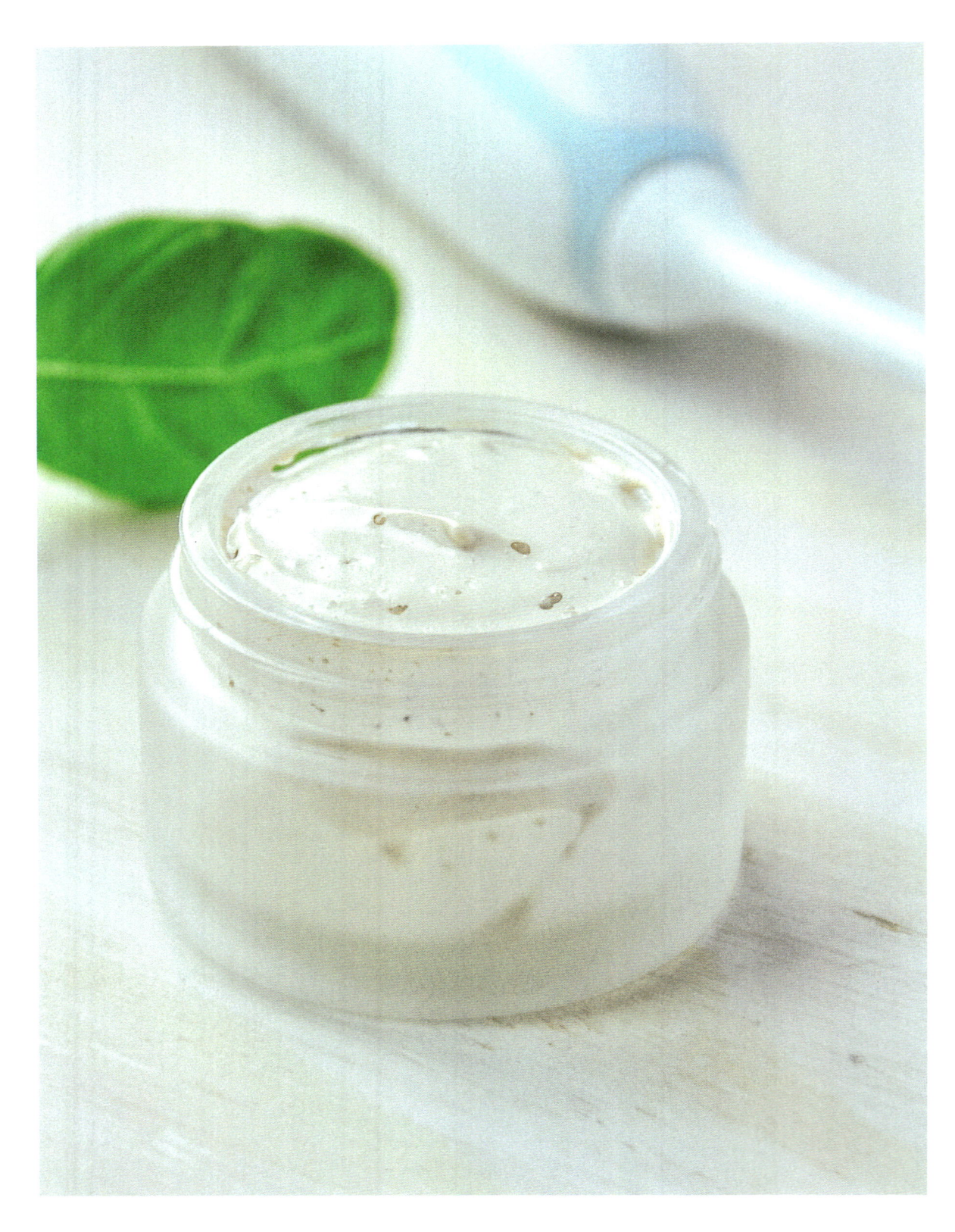

DIY PEPPERMINT TOOTHPASTE

TEETH AND GUM NATURAL CARE

*M*aking homemade toothpaste is cost-effective, easy and works just as well (if not better) than natural store-bought toothpaste. I've created this natural toothpaste recipe with white clay and peppermint essential oil.

White clay or also called Kaolin clay is a mineral-rich clay often used in toothpaste. It is mined all over the world and helps to pull impurities out of the gums and areas surrounding teeth. As an added benefit, white clay has traditionally been used to help aid digestion, so if you swallow some of it, no harm will be done! I like to use A.Vogel clays which are extracted from ancient sea floor deposits and contain natural minerals and trace elements. They are 100% natural, without additives or preservatives.

Bentonite clay is similar to white clay, but it is made from the ash around volcanoes. It is slightly more absorbent than white clay and has natural antibacterial properties. It helps to detoxify heavy metals and removes unhealthy substances from the teeth and gums.

Xylitol is a natural sweetener derived from plant alcohols, most often from corncobs and birch trees. It not only helps to bring a sweet taste to natural toothpaste but naturally disinfects the mouth from bacteria that can lead to tooth decay.

PREP TIME: 10 MINUTES

COOK TIME: 10 MINUTES

TOTAL TIME: 20 MINUTES

MAKES: 10 OZ / 147 ML

INGREDIENTS

- 7 tablespoons of white clay like kaolin or bentonite clay
- 3 tablespoons of mineral water
- 15 drops of peppermint essential oil
- 20 drops of green sweet mint essential oil
- 5 drops of tea tree essential oils or cinnamon essential oils
- 1 teaspoon of coconut oil melted
- 3 teaspoons of xylitol
- 1 teaspoon of baking soda
- 15 drops of grapeseed extract as a natural preservative

INSTRUCTIONS

- Melt the coconut oil if solid in a double boiler
- Once melted, add all the ingredients except the water.
- Once everything is well combined, slowly add the water until it forms a thick paste.
- That's it, you can enjoy brushing your teeth with your new homemade toothpaste!

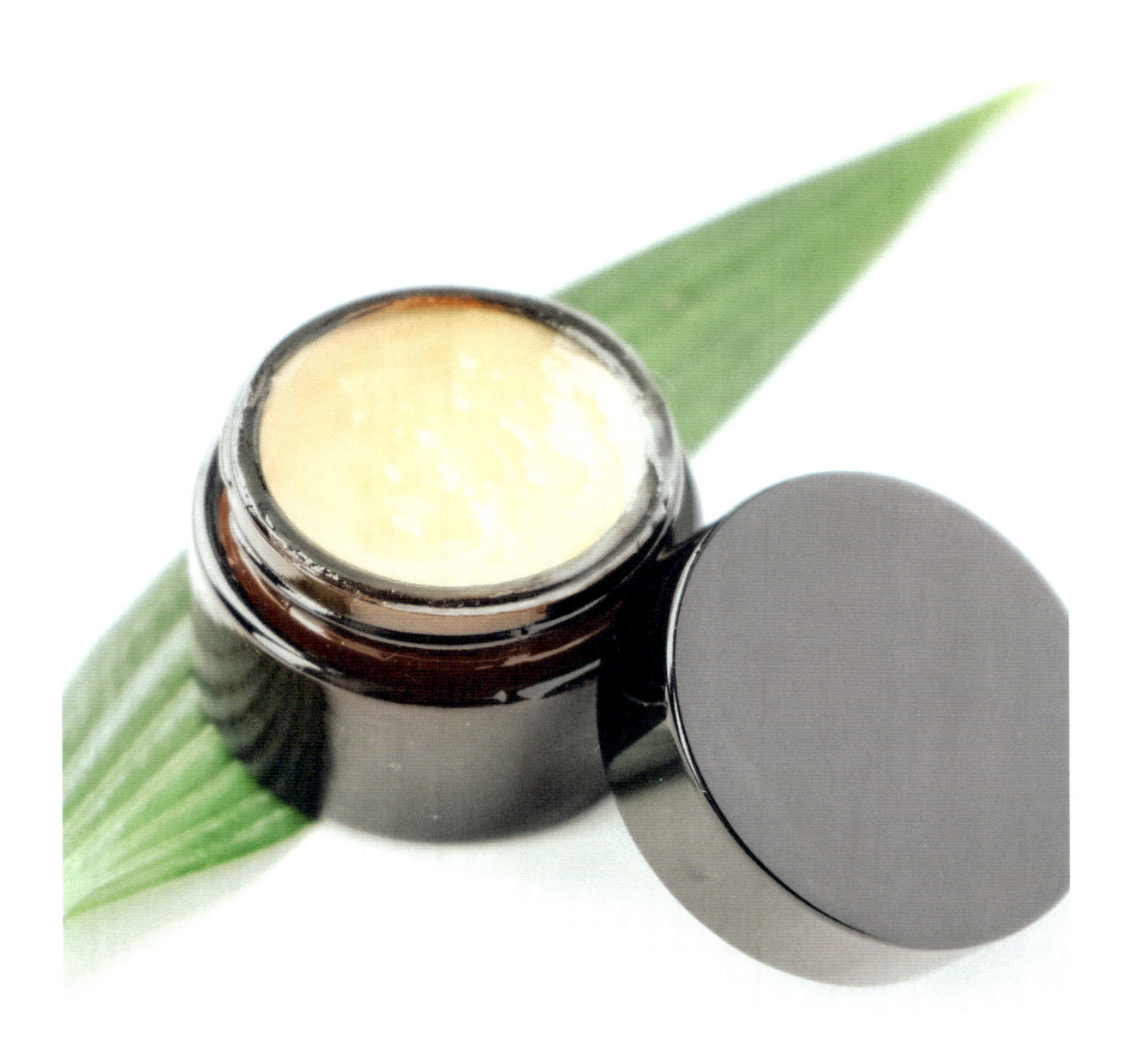

3 DIY FACE BEAUTY PRODUCTS

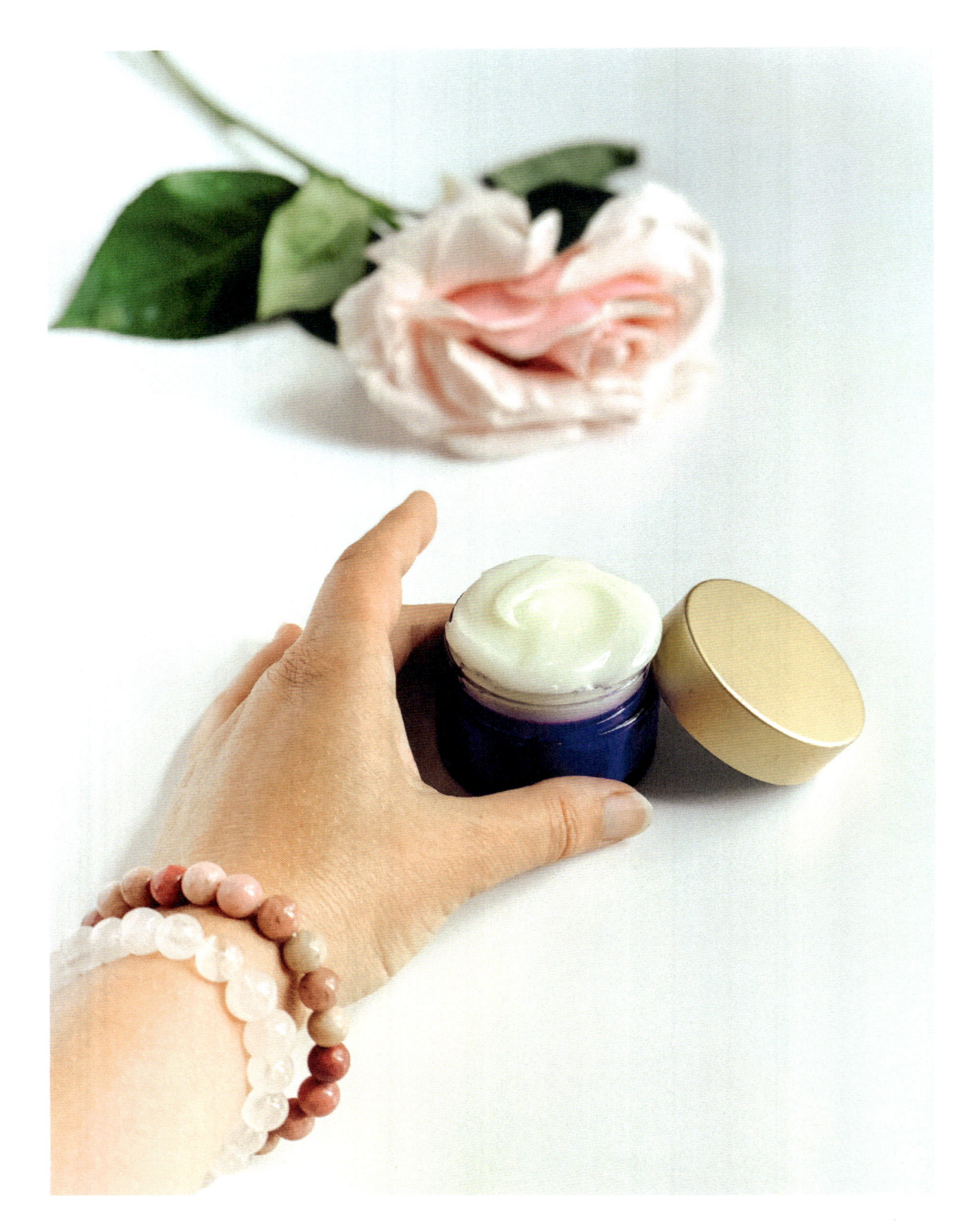

ROSE FACE CREAM

FACE CREAM RECIPES

*T*his Organic face cream recipe is perfect for oily skin or sensitive skins. It is also suitable to all type of skin in the summer when we tend to produce more sebum. Kukui nut oil is definitely one of my favorite oil; I often use it pure and undiluted in the morning on my face.

The great thing about this face cream recipe is that it does not leave a greasy film and absorbs very quickly. For hundreds of years, Hawaiians have used kukui nut oil for its moisturising and healing properties. Lavender; geranium and frankincense essential oils are known to balance the skin and are perfect for oily skin... needless to say the rose scent is heavenly!

PREP TIME: 15 MINUTES

COOK TIME: 10 MINUTES

TOTAL TIME: 25 MINUTES

MAKES: 1.6 OZ / 47 ML

INGREDIENTS

- 2 teaspoons of organic rose flower water (You can substitute with lemongrass or Lavender hydrosols)
- 7 teaspoons of organic kukui nut oil
- 0.5 teaspoon of natural white beeswax pellets (or yellow)
- 5 drops of organic Lavender essential oil
- 5 drops of organic rose Geranium essential oil
- 5 drops of organic frankincense essential oil
- 1 drop of organic grapeseed extract
- Glass Salve Containers

INSTRUCTIONS

- Combine the oils & beeswax in your double boiler on low heat.
- At the same time, add the rose water in another double boiler on low heat so that it gets to the same temperatures as the oils.
- Once the oils are melted, take it off the heat and start whipping with an electric or manual mixer fast.
- Add the rose water drop by drop while mixing. Do not stop mixing!
- Continue mixing until you reach the creamy consistency desired for 2 to 5 minutes.
- If you are having trouble creating the emulsifier, add your recipient in another bowl filled of cold (not iced) water. Be sure to starting mixing right away and not to splash any water in the cream.
- Add the essential oils and mix well.
- Use within 2 months!

100   ORGANIC BEAUTY RECIPES BY EVE

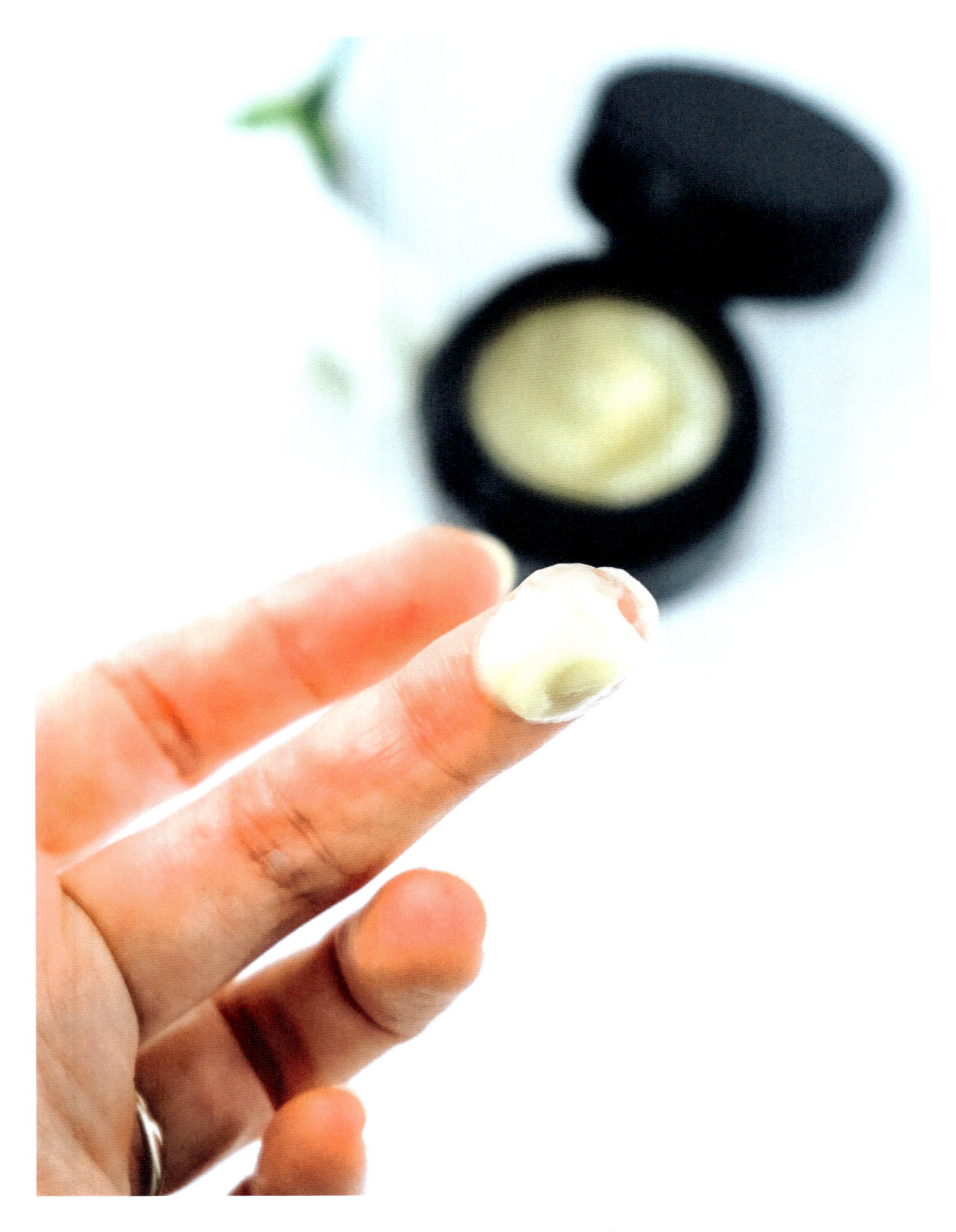

FACE MOISTURIZER WITH ROYAL JELLY

FACE CREAM RECIPES

After lots of research and experiments, I have created with my own version of a face moisturizer with Royal Jelly, a similar version of the "famous" Egyptian magic cream with jojoba oil, orange blossom hydrosol, bee propolis, royal jelly and beeswax. It works wonders for fine lines, wrinkles and as a homemade eye cream treatment.

Royal Jelly Powder Dried & Frozen

Royal jelly, a secretion from the glands of worker bees and is fed to the larvae. It offers numerous skin benefits that include:
- Anti-inflammatory properties
- Improves skin texture
- Reduces the appearance of dark circles
- Reduces dark spots and scars
- Treats acne
- Fights Candida, Eczema etc.

Royal Jelly is a powerful skin ingredient that can help you achieve flawless skin. It helps in smoothening out your wrinkles and adds a youthful touch to the skin, making it glow. You can get dried freeze royal jelly powder online on amazon.

Bee Propolis Extract

More commonly referred to as bee glue, bee propolis that the honeybees produce by mixing beeswax and saliva with exudate gathered from sap flows, tree buds and other sources (botanical). While bees primarily harvest nectar and pollen, they also collect tree resin and water for making Propolis to glue the small gaps present in a hive.

Bee Propolis extract benefits:
- Reduce inflammation and redness
- Reduce pigmentation
- Boost collagen production
- Offer antioxidant protection against sunlight, radiation, and pollution

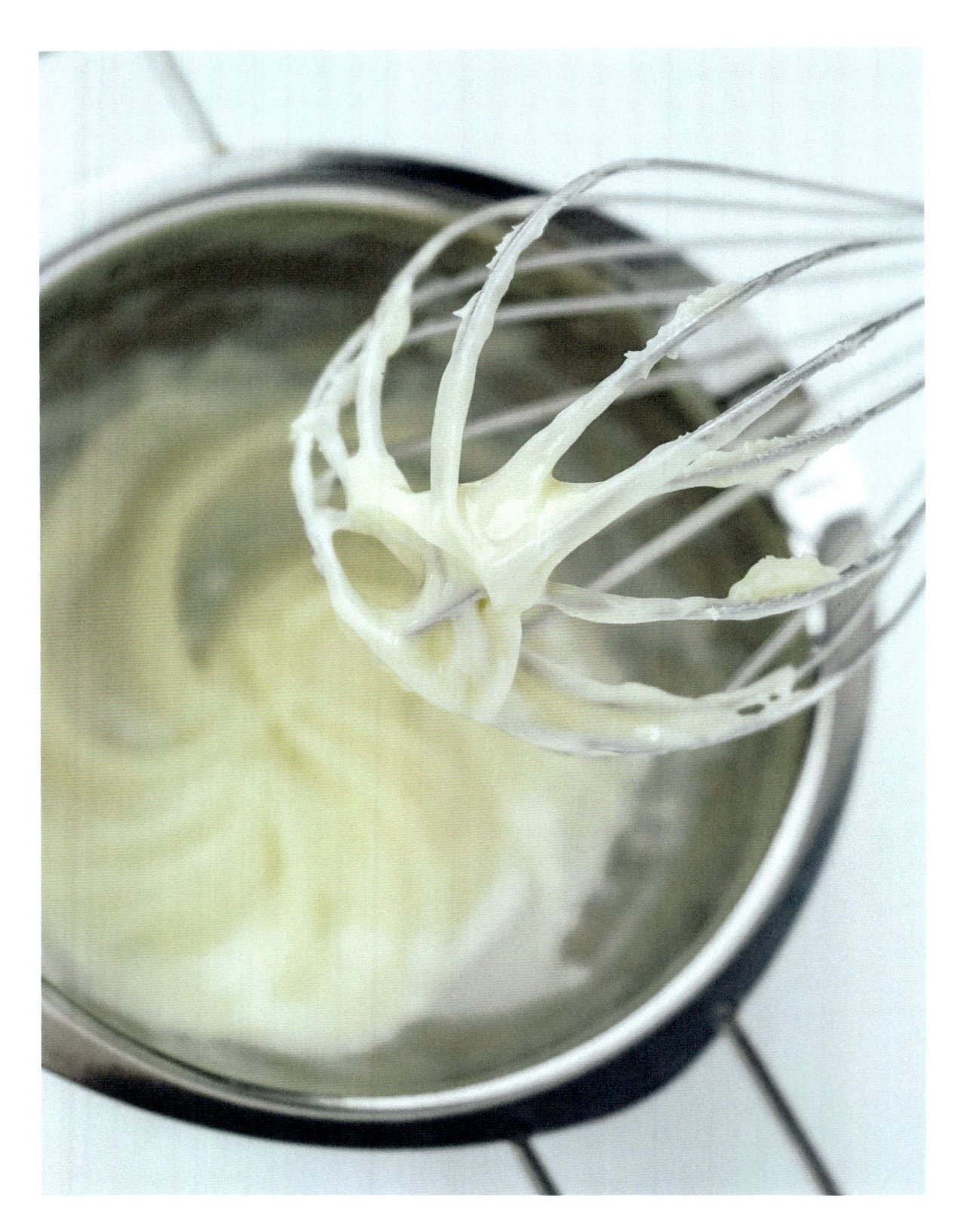

FACE MOISTURIZER WITH ROYAL JELLY

FACE CREAM RECIPES

PREP TIME: 10 MINUTES

COOK TIME: 10 MINUTES

TOTAL TIME: 20 MINUTES

MAKES: 1.6 OZ / 47 ML

INGREDIENTS

- 7 teaspoons organic jojoba oil
- 1 teaspoons orange blossom hydrosol
- 1 teaspoon white beeswax pellets
- ½ teaspoon dried freezed royal gelly powder
- 5 drops bee propolis extract (liquid)
- 5 drops lavender essential oil
- 1 drop of grapeseed extract as a natural preservative

INSTRUCTIONS

- Add the white beeswax, jojoba oil and orange blossom a double boiler or an aluminum bowl filled with water on medium-high heat, until they are melted.
- Remove from the heat and immediately mix with a manual egg beater spatula until the cream starts to form and until it is the consistency of a cream. Your spatula must leave marks in the cream.
- Add the dried freeze royal jelly powder, mix well.
- Add the bee propolis, mix well.
- Add the lavender essential oil and grapeseed extract and mix well.
- Pour in a glass jar container. It's best to keep this cream in the fridge to keep the properties of the dried freeze royal jelly intact.
- Apply at night, before going to bed like a cold cream.

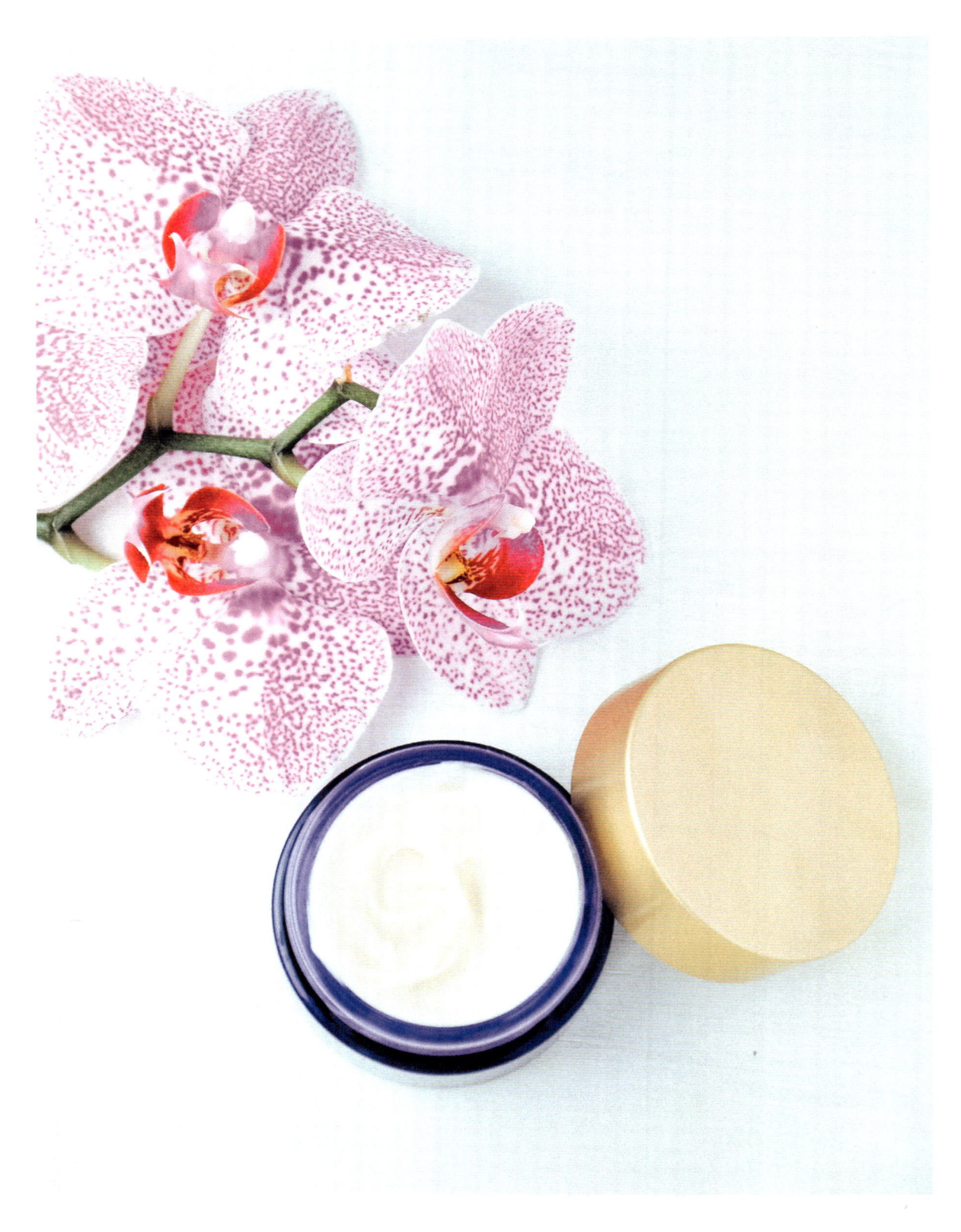

FACE CREAM WITH SACHA INCHI OIL FOR MATURE SKIN

FACE CREAM RECIPES

I am always on the lookout for rare carrier oils that I can experiment with for new recipes! Sacha inchi oil comes from a plant native to South America and parts of the Caribbean. The seeds of the sacha inchi tree slightly resemble peanuts – the oil produced from the seeds is edible and used in cooking – but, it also has amazing benefits for skin and hair!

PREP TIME: 10 MINUTES

TOTAL TIME: 10 MINUTES

MAKES: 17 OZ / 500 ML

INGREDIENTS

- 1 cup of refined shea butter
- 1 cup of sacha inchi oil
- 4 tablespoons of chamomile hydrosol
- 20 drops of lavender essential oil
- 10 drops of rose geranium essential oil
- 5 drops of frankincense essential oil
- 5 drops of grapeseed extract as a natural preservative

INSTRUCTIONS

- Add the shea butter and sacha inchi oil in an aluminum bowl.
- Mix the shea butter and sacha inchi oil with a hand blender until smooth.
- Add the 4 tablespoons of the chamomile flower water one spoon at a time and mix well with the hand blender until smooth and well combined for at least 5 minutes.
- Pour the cream into glass containers.
- The cream will become thicker as it sets after a few hours. It will remain soft to the touch which makes this homemade face cream easy to apply.

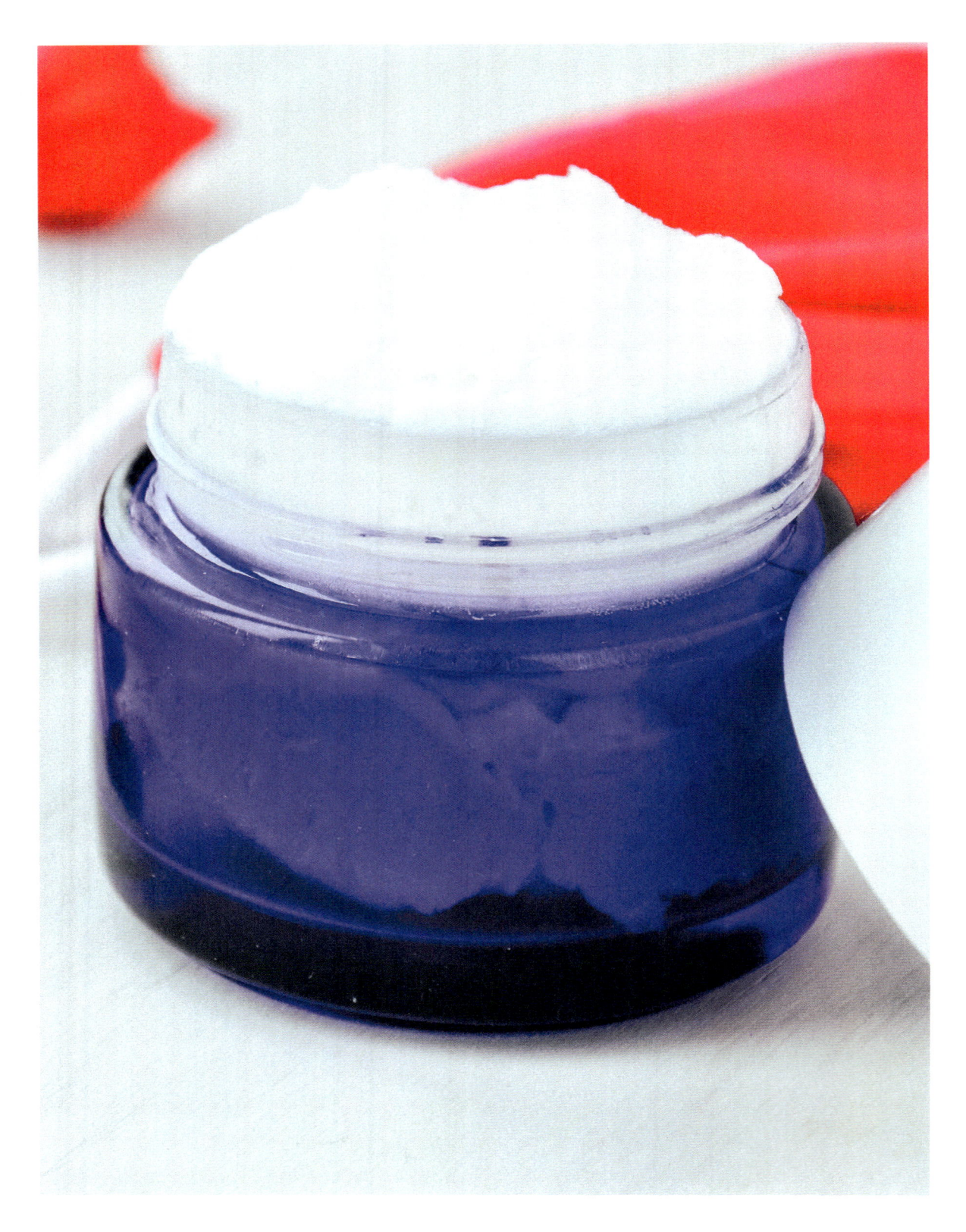

DIY MAKE UP REMOVER CREAM

FACE CREAM RECIPES

*M*aking your own DIY eye makeup remover is super easy and requires 3 ingredients: shea butter, camellia seed oil and chamomile flower water (hydrosol) and can be done in 5 to 10 minutes.

PREP TIME: 10 MINUTES

TOTAL TIME: 10 MINUTES

MAKES: 17 OZ / 500 ML

INGREDIENTS

- 12 tablespoons of shea butter
- 8 tablespoons of camelia seed oil
- 2 tablespoons of chamomile hydrosol
- 30 drops of grapeseed extract as a natural preservative

INSTRUCTIONS

- Add the shea butter and camelia seed oil in an aluminum bowl.
- Mix the shea butter and camelia seed oil with a hand blender until smooth.
- Add the 2 tablespoons of the chamomile flower water one spoon at a time and mix well with the hand blender until smooth and well combined. You will have a smooth cream, like a lotion.
- Add the natural preservative, mix well.
- Pour the cream into glass containers. The cream will become thicker as it sets after a few hours.
- Use a 2 cotton pad and apply the cream to your closed eyelids, wiping and patting gently until all eye makeup is removed.

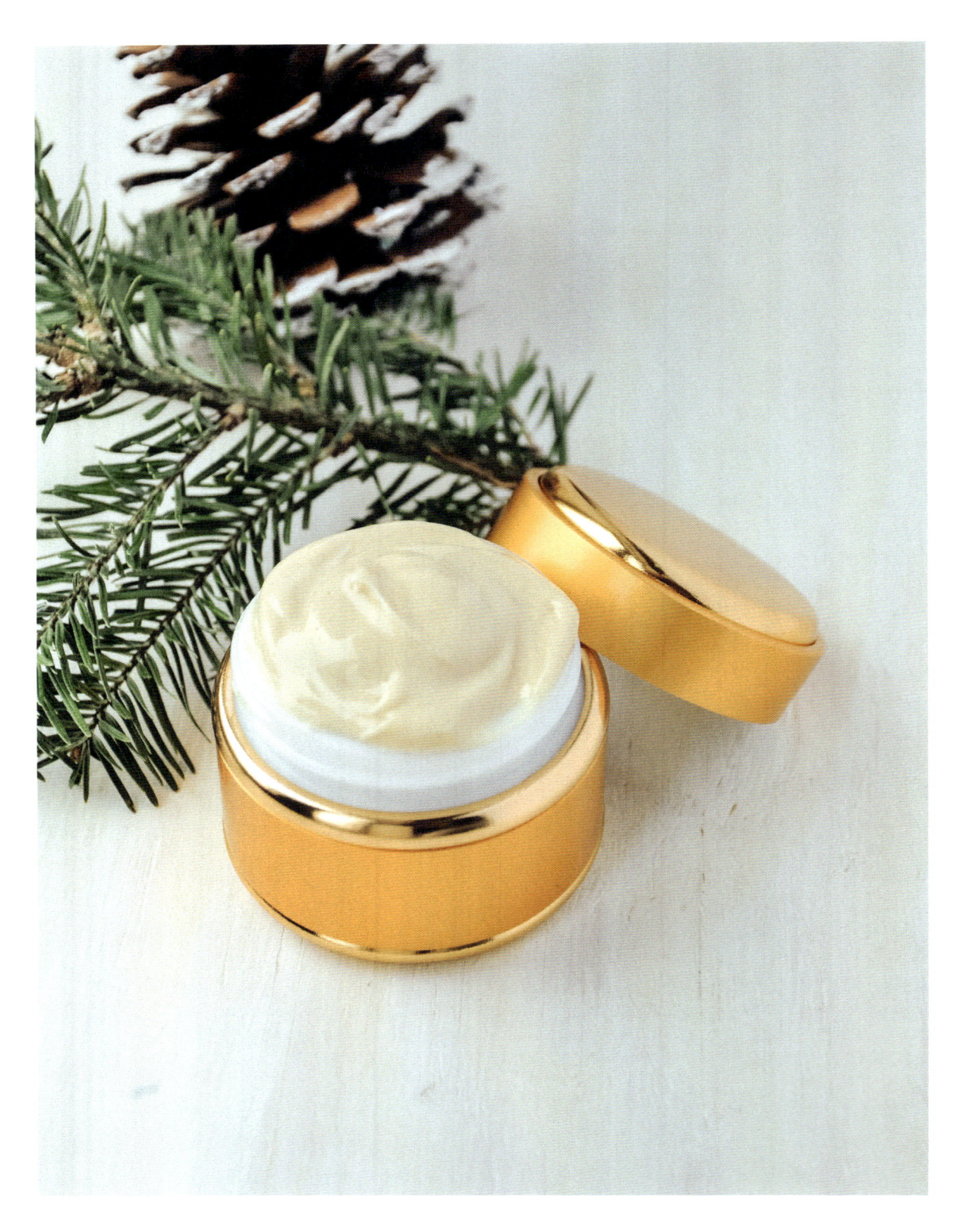

ANTI AGING FACE CREAM WITHOUT BEESWAX

FACE CREAM RECIPES

I used my homemade anti-aging cream with Uccuba butter, argan oil, shea butter and camelia seed oil for two months now and have noticed a difference in the appearance of my skin: less fine lines, more even tone, and it's also helping to keep my acne at bay!

The best part of this DIY anti-wrinkle recipe is that there is no beeswax. I've also used a blend of essential oils that helps fight the signs of aging on your face.

PREP TIME: 30 MINUTES

COOK TIME: 10 MINUTES

TOTAL TIME: 40 MINUTES

MAKES: 2.5 OZ / 73 ML

INGREDIENTS

- 3 tablespoons of uccuba butter
- 1 tablespoon of shea butter
- 3 tablespoons of argan oil
- 5 tablespoons of camelia seed oil
- 5 drops of frankincense essential oil
- 5 drops of rose geranium essential oil
- 5 drops of ho wood essential oil

INSTRUCTIONS

- Melt the uccuba butter and shea butter in a double boiler.
- Once melted, add the argan and camelia seed oil.
- Mix well.
- Put the recipient in the freezer for 15-20 mins, until the ingredients have hardened but are not completely frozen.
- Take it out of the freezer and start mixing with a hand blender until it is nice and creamy.
- Add the essential oils if you wish.
- Pour into nice containers.
- Voila, you have made your own homemade anti-aging cream recipe!

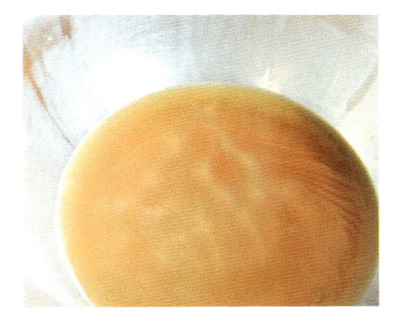

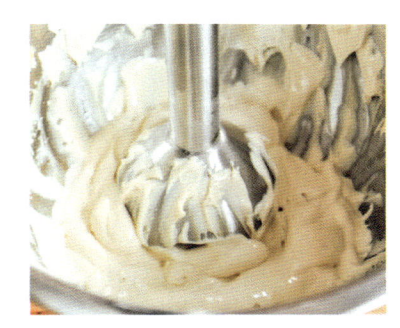

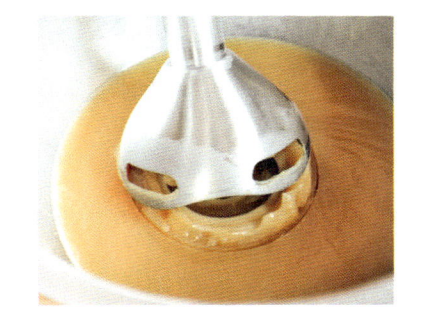

ORGANIC BEAUTY RECIPES BY EVE

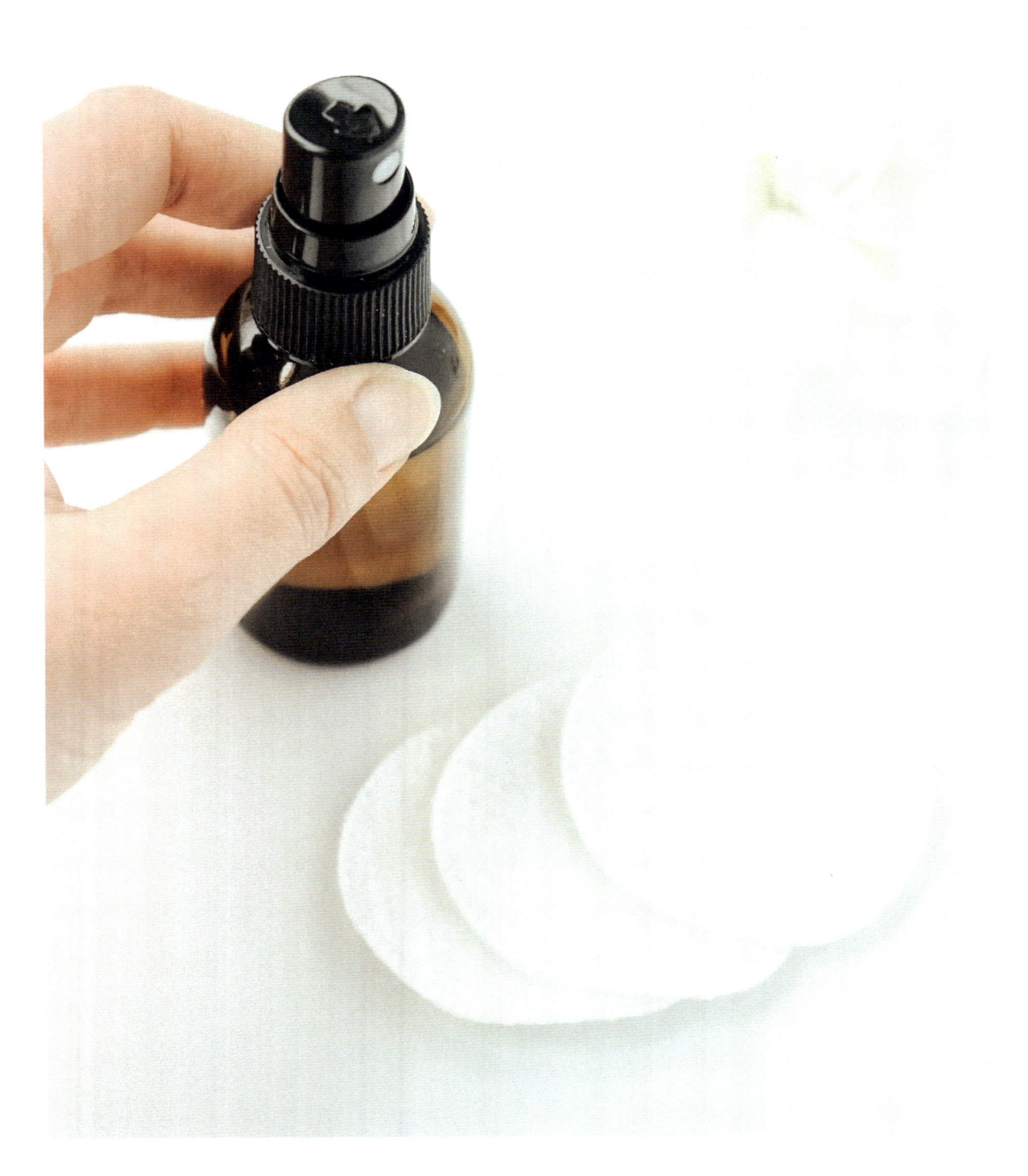

OIL CLEANSING METHOD FOR ACNE

FACE SERUM

*H*ave you ever heard of the oil cleansing method for acne and wondered what that is? Are you wondering why you would put oil on your face if you already have oily skin? The last thing you would want on your face is more oil, right? Think again!

Even though the words oil, cleansing, and acne seem like complete misfits, you'd be amazed by the way things would turn out for you if you took my advice and followed this simple daily skincare routine to get clear acne-free skin.

My favorite face oils are jojoba oil, followed by rosehip oil and camelia seed oil!

What is the OCM Method?

The OCM method (short for oil cleansing method) is simply using pure oils to clean your skin or impurities and hydrate it at the same time.

Benefits of the Oil Cleansing Method for Acne

Here are 4 reasons why you should use the oil cleansing method for acne:

- It is completely organic and does not use any harmful chemicals
- It preserves your skin's natural oils
- Very simple routine and it's quite easy to make
- Does not even cost a lot of money

PREP TIME: 5 MINUTES

TOTAL TIME: 5 MINUTES

MAKES: 1 OZ / 30 ML

INGREDIENTS

- 30 ml of organic jojoba oil
- 30 ml of rose or orange blossom hydrosol
- 30 ml of Rosehip oil (optional)

INSTRUCTIONS

- Gather some cotton pads, jojoba oil, and some lukewarm water.
- Clean your face and remove your makeup using rose hydrosol or orange blossom hydrosol. This will prep your skin for the next crucial step.
- Add a few drops of jojoba oil on the cotton pad to help remove traces of dirt.
- After your face is clean, take a few drops of Jojoba oil and massage your face gently for a few minutes.
- If you would like you can also add a few drops of rosehip oil for anti-aging properties. And you're done!
- Now leave that oil on your face overnight.
- This will also act as a moisturizer and night cream. No need to add an extra layer of moisturizer -Remember, less is more!

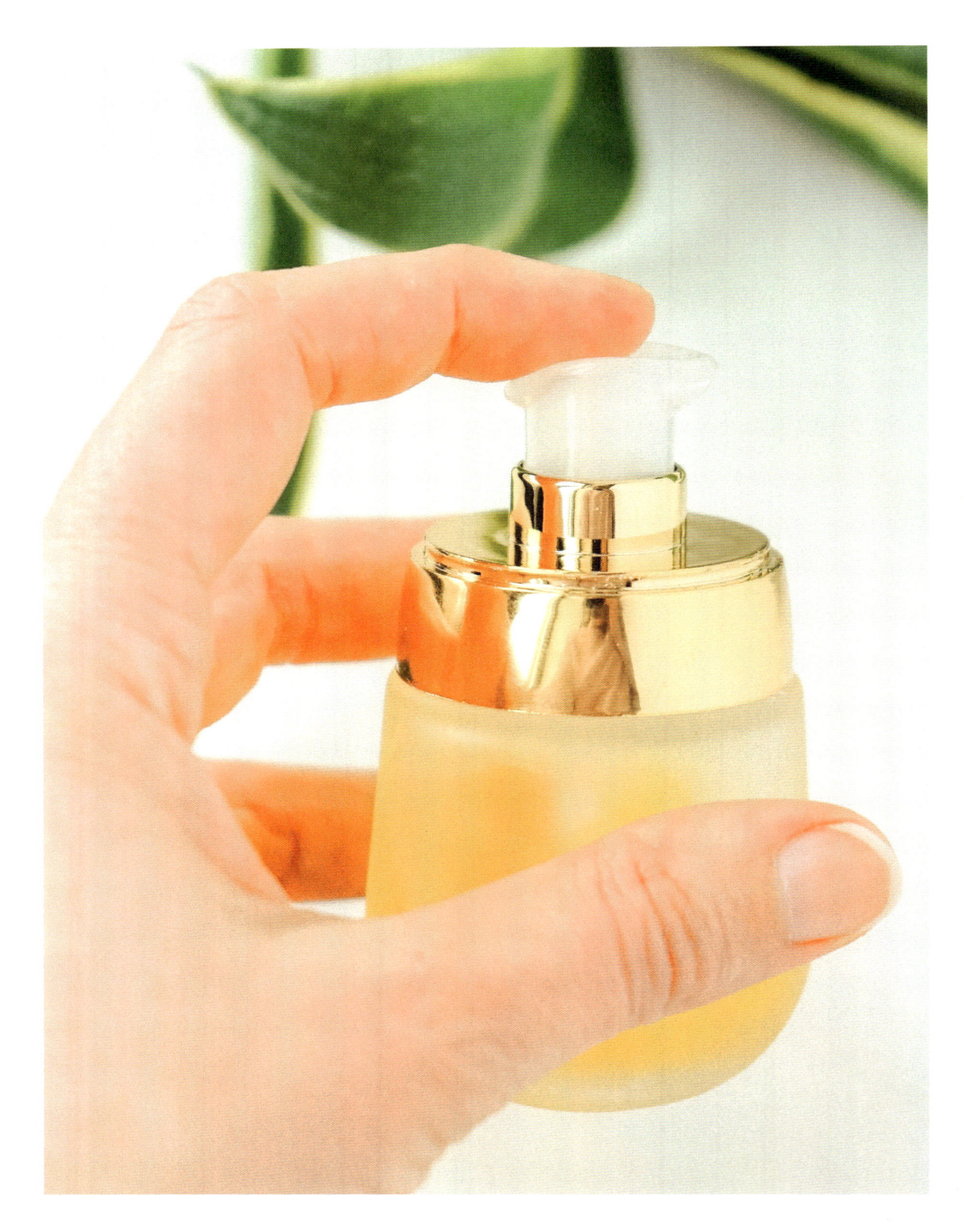

HOMEMADE FACE SERUM FOR OILY SKIN

FACE SERUM

I have formulated this natural homemade face serum recipe that is easy to make and can also be customized to your skin type. This is much cheaper when compared to the store-bought expensive serums and skin transformation creams. Because you can buy these oils wholesale online, they will cost you a fraction of the cost!

PREP TIME: 5 MINUTES

TOTAL TIME: 5 MINUTES

MAKES: 1 OZ / 30 ML

INGREDIENTS

- 1 tablespoon of jojoba oil
- 1 tablespoon of grapeseed oil
- 4 drops of Ylang Ylang Essential Oil
- 4 drops of Lavender Essential Oil
- 4 drops of Patchouli Essential Oil
- 1 30ml 1oz Empty Refillable Glass Container Pump Bottle

INSTRUCTIONS

- Pour all the ingredients together in a glass container and shake well.
- Apply and massage 3 to 4 drops or 1 pump on your clean face every morning and evening.
- Use within 6 months.

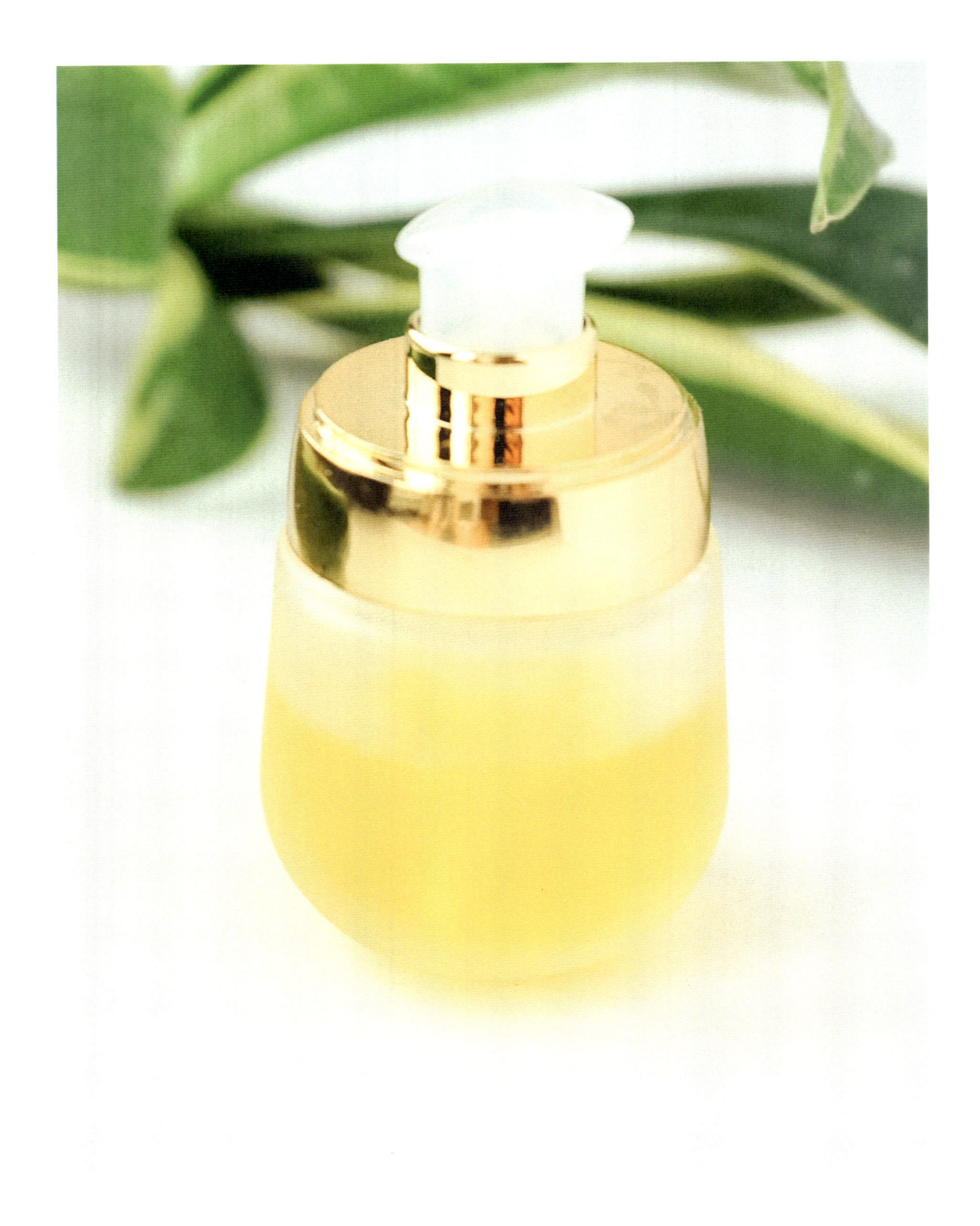

HOMEMADE FACE SERUM FOR DRY SKIN

FACE SERUM

*I*n this simple yet effective homemade face serum, I have used jojoba oil and argan oil.

Jojoba Oil
Helps moisturize the skin and reduces dry patches. It contains sebum that oily skin generates naturally, hence lubricating dry skin.

Argan Oil
The high fatty acid and vitamin E content boosts hydration and softens dry skin.

PREP TIME: 5 MINUTES

TOTAL TIME: 5 MINUTES

MAKES: 1 OZ - 30 ML

INGREDIENTS

- 1 and 1/2 tablespoons of jojoba oil
- 1/2 tablespoon of argan oil
- 4 drops Palmarosa Essential Oil
- 4 drops Roman Or German Chamomile Essential Oil
- 4 drops Lavender Essential Oil
- 1 30 ml 1oz Empty Refillable Glass Container Pump Bottle

INSTRUCTIONS

- Pour all the ingredients together in a glass container and shake well.
- Apply and massage 3 to 4 drops or 1 pump on your clean face every morning and evening.
- Use within 6 months.

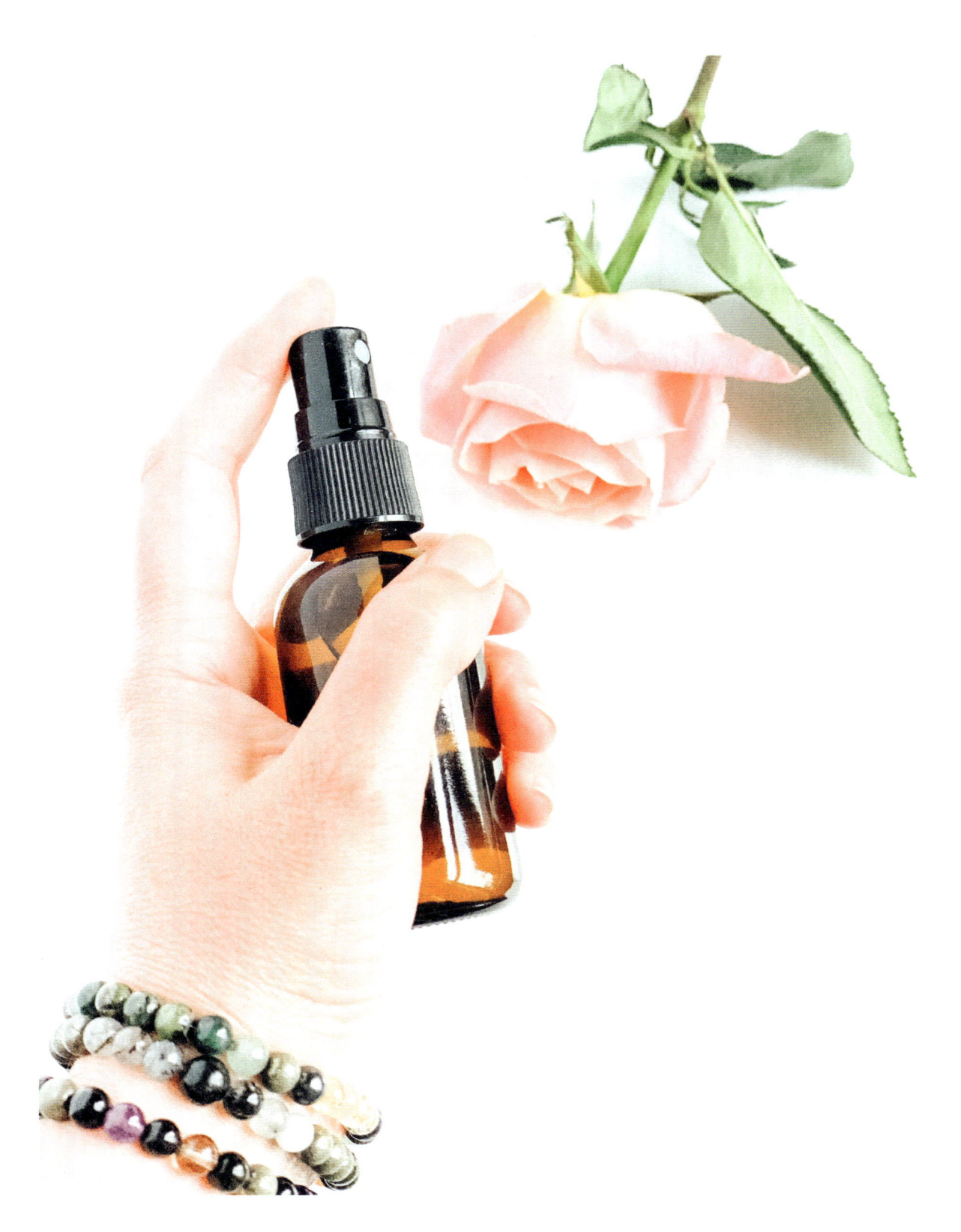

DIY FACE SERUM RECIPE ANTI WRINKLES

FACE SERUM

If you are looking for a simple and natural way of taking care of your face while preventing the appearance of fine lines, you should make this easy DIY face serum recipe. It's as easy as blending organic rosehip oil and essential oils together!

There is no need to heat up anything, nor even create an emulsion. Just pour the rosehip oil and essential oils, shake it and use it!

PREP TIME: 5 MINUTES

TOTAL TIME: 5 MINUTES

MAKES: 1 OZ OR 30 ML

INGREDIENTS
- 2 tablespoons of organic rosehip oil
- 5 drops of essential oil of rose geranium
- 2 drops of lavender essential oil
- 2 drops of frankincense essential oil
- 1 drops of sandalwood essential oil optional
- 1 drops of carrot seed essential oil
- 2 drops of helichrysum essential oil
- 1 glass amber bottle with eye dropper or blue cobalt glass bottle with eye dropper OR
- 1 glass cobalt boston round with black pump

INSTRUCTIONS

- Pour all the ingredients together in a dark glass container and shake well.
- Apply and massage 4 to 5 drops or 1 pump on your clean face every morning and evening.
- Use within 6 months.

How long until I see the result of reducing wrinkles on my skin?
You should use it twice a day, morning and evening for at least 2 weeks to min a month to see the results on your face.

I've been using this face oil recipe for years and it's my secret weapon when I want clear and smooth skin.

My face is acne prone and this diy face serum recipe helps to prevent pimples and heals my skin fast. It helps reducing dark spots and fine lines due to sun damage. I also love the natural glow and tan effect it gives me!

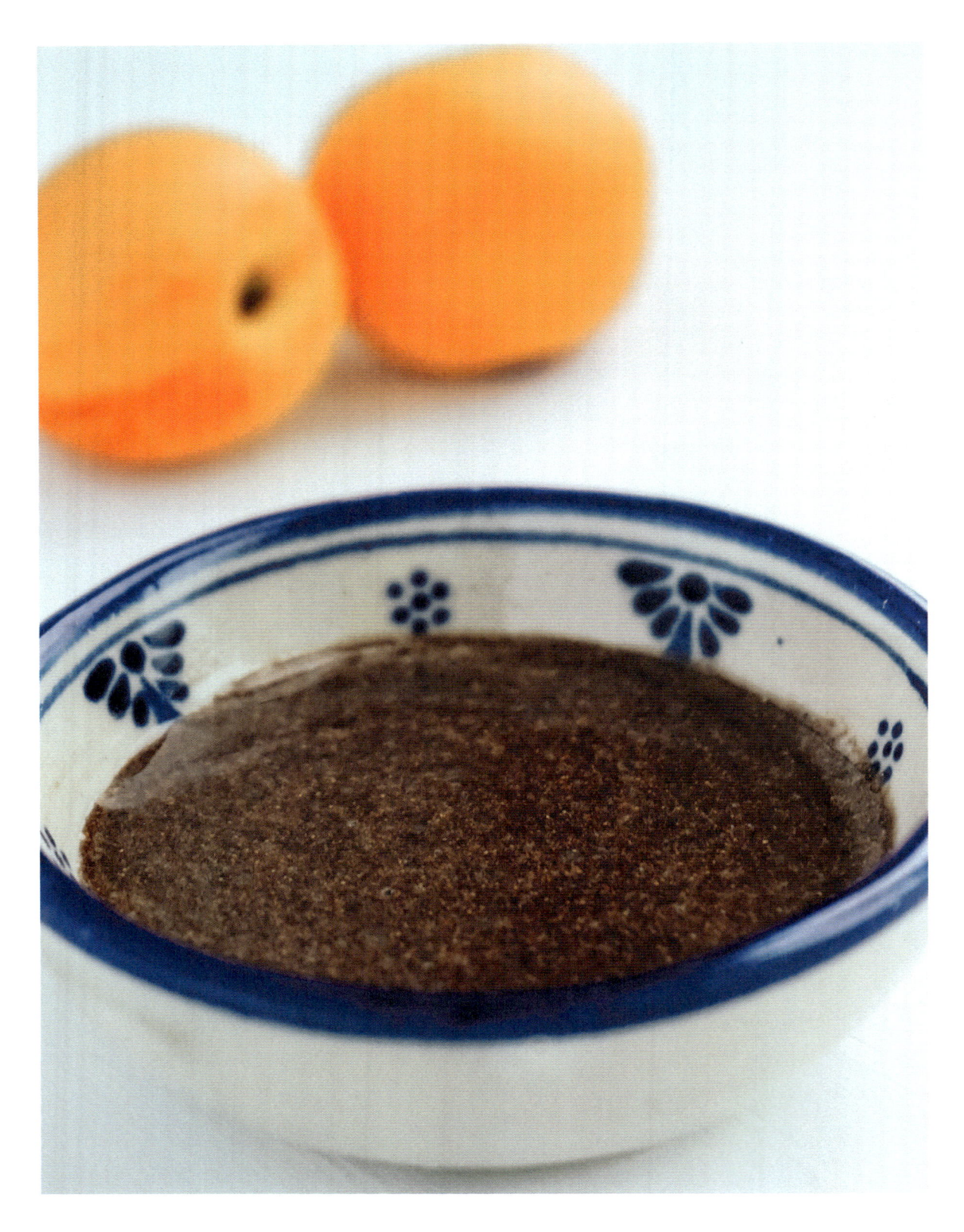

FACE SCRUB WITH APRICOT KERNEL POWDER

FACE SCRUBS

Forget about your pricey so called high-end face scrubs full of chemicals, I'm going to teach how to make an easy face scrub with apricot kernel powder at home. Apricot kernel powder is such a perfect ingredient because of its amazing exfoliating benefits on the skin. I've also used maple syrup and Rhassoul clay (Moroccan clay) to draw the impurities out of your face. It is suitable for all type of skins.

PREP TIME: 10 MINUTES

TOTAL TIME: 10 MINUTES

MAKES: ONE APPLICATION

INGREDIENTS
- 2 teaspoons of Apricot kernel powder
- 1 teaspoon of Rhassoul clay
- 3 teaspoons of maple syrup

INSTRUCTIONS

- Start by grinding the apricot kernels in a fast blender if you bought the actual apricot kernel. You need to reduce it to a fine powder. I suggest you use a Vitamix or a ninja blender. It needs to be powerful enough to grind really hard nuts! If you managed to find apricot kernel powder, then of course not need to grind it.
- Sift the apricot kernel powder with a sieve.
- Mix all the ingredients into a small bowl until they are well integrated. You may opt to whisk them, but just folding them in with a spatula will do.
- Apply directly to the face and massage gently for a few minutes in small circular motions.
- Rinse well with lukewarm water and apply your daily moisturizer.
- You may store the leftovers in a small container for a few weeks as long as there is no contamination with water.

120   ORGANIC BEAUTY RECIPES BY EVE

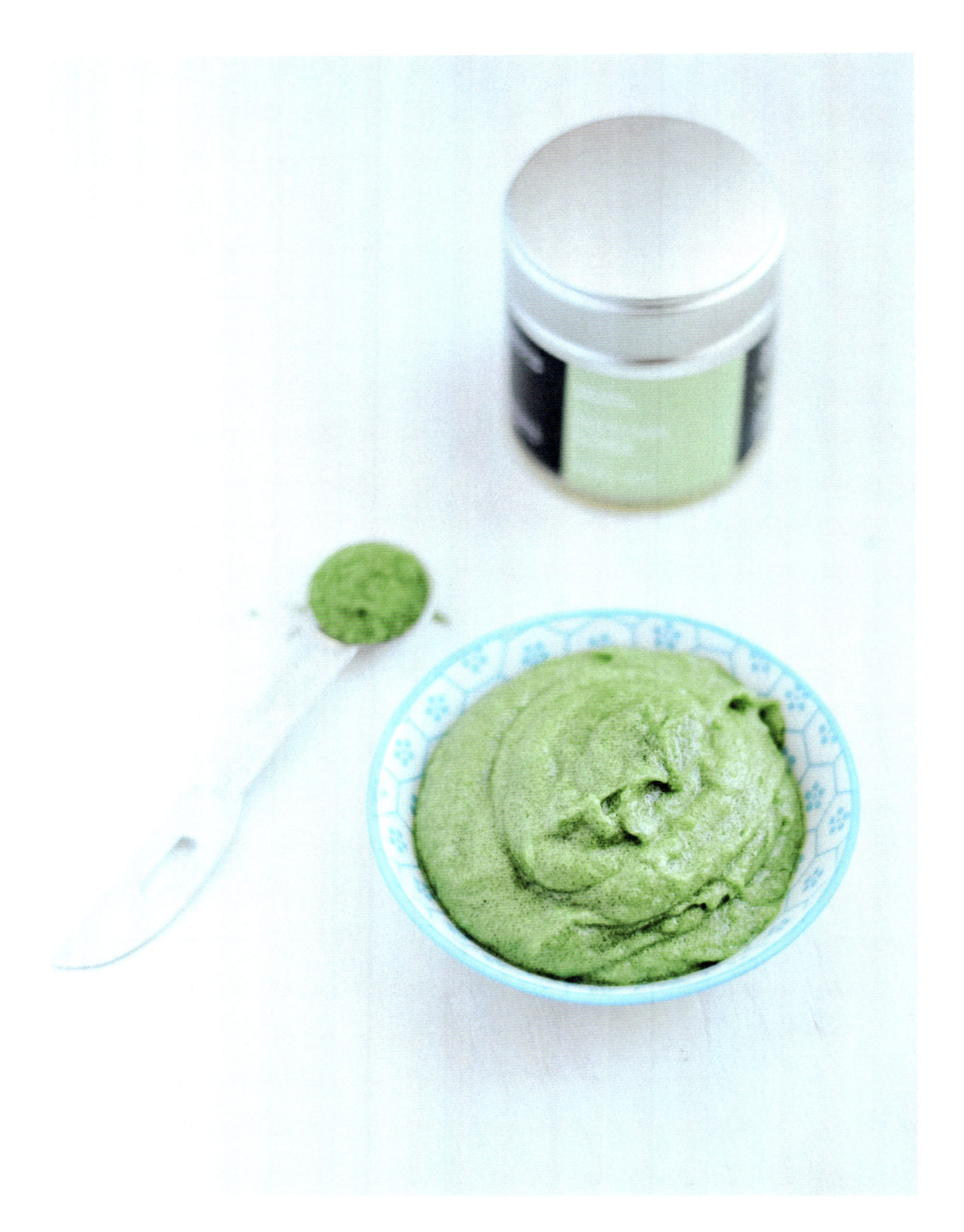

MATCHA SUGAR SCRUB

FACE SCRUBS

Attention to all tea addicts! Did you know that the benefits of matcha on skin are plenty?

This matcha sugar scrub recipe does wonders for your skin. It is a great detoxifier and will make your skin glow. It also helps to repair the effect of aging.

PREP TIME: 10 MINUTES

TOTAL TIME: 10 MINUTES

MAKES: 16 OZ / 500 ML

INGREDIENTS

- 1 teaspoon of matcha green tea
- ½ cup of organic non refined coconut oil
- ¼ cup of organic safflower oil
- 1 cup + ½ cup of organic sugar refined

INSTRUCTIONS

- Whip the coconut oil for a minute or two until it is creamy. It needs to be solidifies so you can whip it. If it is melted (usually around 25C), put it in the fridge for 1 hour.
- Add the oil and continue whipping.
- Add the sugar, matcha and mix well.
- Finally add the essential oils.
- Pour in pretty jars.
- This will last a month since there is no water. It is best to keep it in the fridge so the sugar does not dissolve with the oils.
- Always take care of using a clean spoon to scoop the scrub so you don't contaminate it.
- Gently scrub your face once a week.
- Rinse well with warm water.

Word of caution
If you have never used matcha on your skin before, it's always best to do a patch test in case you have an allergic reaction. Better be safe than sorry!

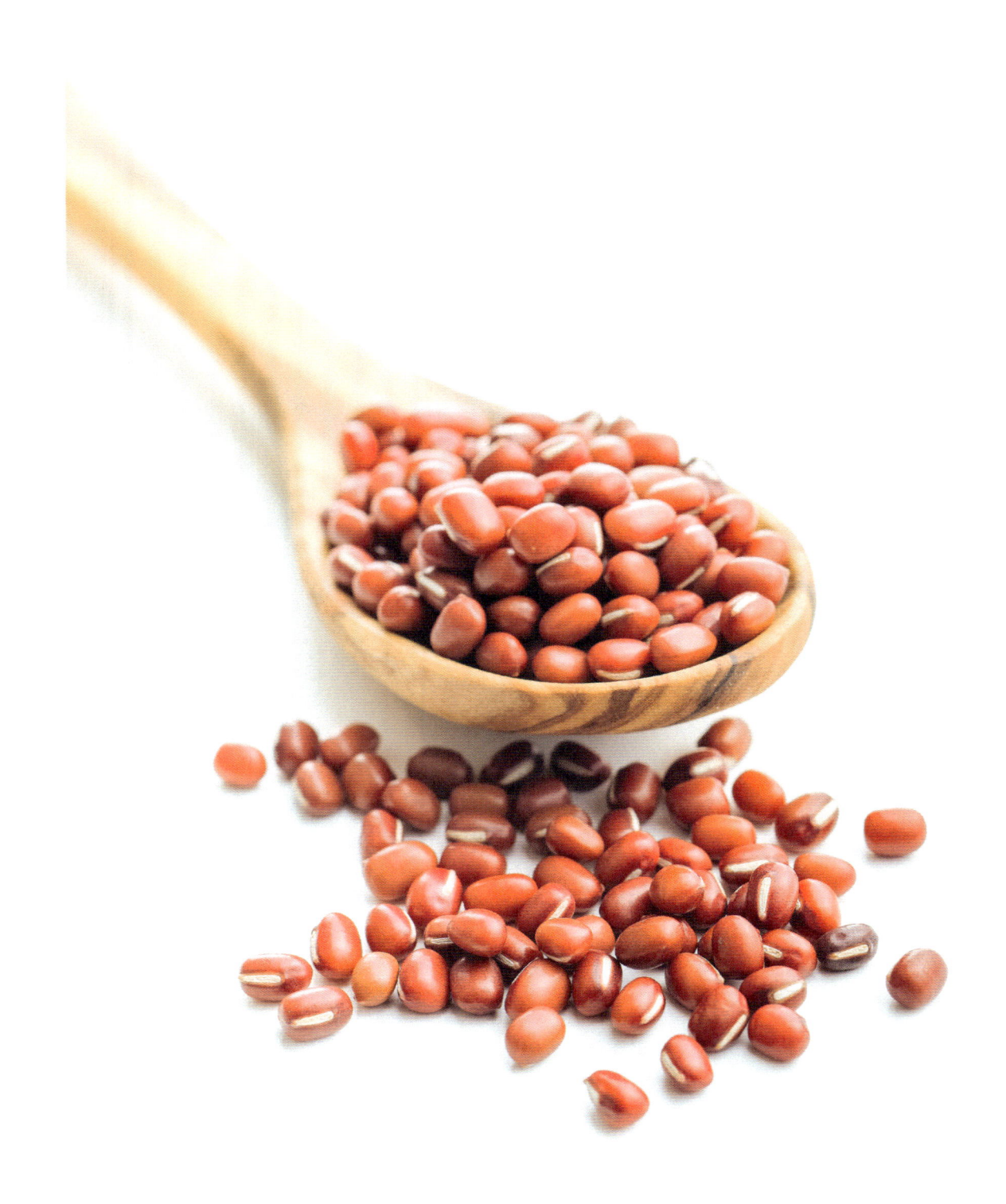

ADZUKI BEAN FACE SCRUB

FACE SCRUBS

Who would not trust Japanese women for their traditional ways of taking care of their beautiful and flawless skin? One of their ancient secrets is the adzuki bean (also called azuki beans) which, when ground and made into a scrub, gently exfoliates and removes dull skin.

I happened to have some organic adzuki beans left over in my pantry and I was looking for a new kind of face scrub. It's amazing how many DIY beauty products come from what you might have in your kitchen! This is a very simple, easy and cost efficient way of making a homemade face scrub. All you need is azuki beans and a powerful blender to grind the beans like Ninja or Vitamix.

PREP TIME: 10 MINUTES

TOTAL TIME: 10 MINUTES

MAKES: SEVERAL APPLICATIONS - DO NOT MIX WITH WATER UNTIL YOU ARE READY TO USE.

INGREDIENTS

- 1 cup of dried organic azuki beans
- Coffee grinder or your favorite fast speed blender like Ninja or Vitamix
- Mineral water or aloe vera juice enough to form a thick paste.
- Sieve optional

INSTRUCTIONS

- Grind the adzuki beans in your fast-speed blender until they are completely ground like coarse flour.
- Sift the adzuki flour with a sieve to remove the biggest chunks of the beans if necessary.
- Pour in an airtight glass container.
- You should have enough powder for several applications.

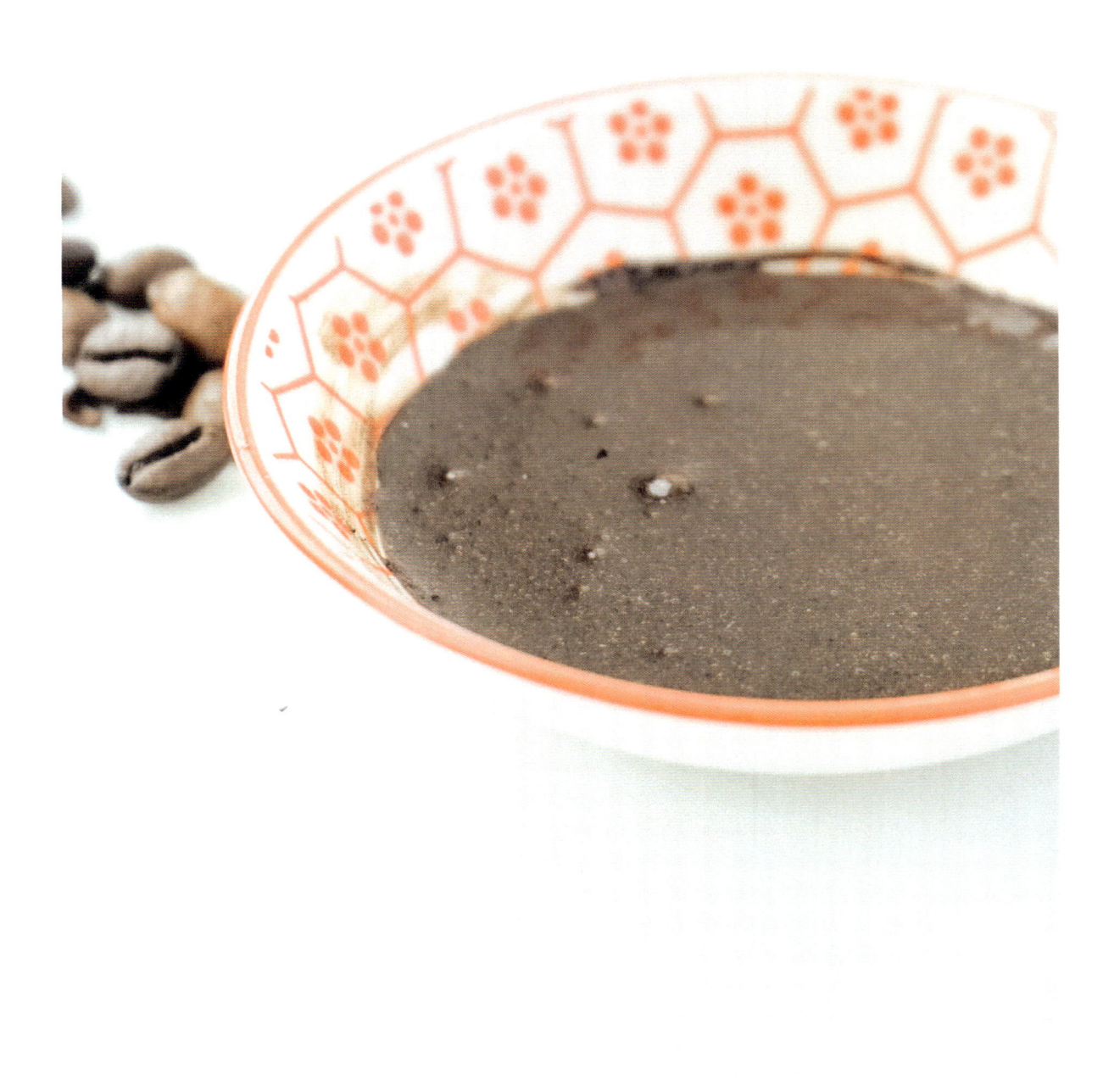

COFFEE FACE SCRUB RECIPE

FACE SCRUBS

*M*y coffee face scrub recipe is easy to make with only 3 ingredients: coffee, kaolin clay, and organic agave nectar.

PREP TIME: 10 MINUTES

TOTAL TIME: 10 MINUTES

MAKES: ONE APPLICATION

INGREDIENTS

- 2 teaspoons of agave nectar or maple syrup
- 2 teaspoons of ground coffee beans
- 1 teaspoons of kaolin clay

INSTRUCTIONS

- Mix all the ingredients into a small bowl until they are well integrated. You may opt to whisk them, but just folding them in with a spatula will do.
- Apply directly to the face and massage gently for a few minutes in small circular motions.
- Rinse well with lukewarm water and apply your daily DIY moisturizer.
- You may store the leftovers in a small container for a few weeks as long as there is no contamination with water.

Word of caution

If you have never used coffee on your skin before, it's always best to do a patch test in case you have an allergic reaction. Better be safe than sorry!

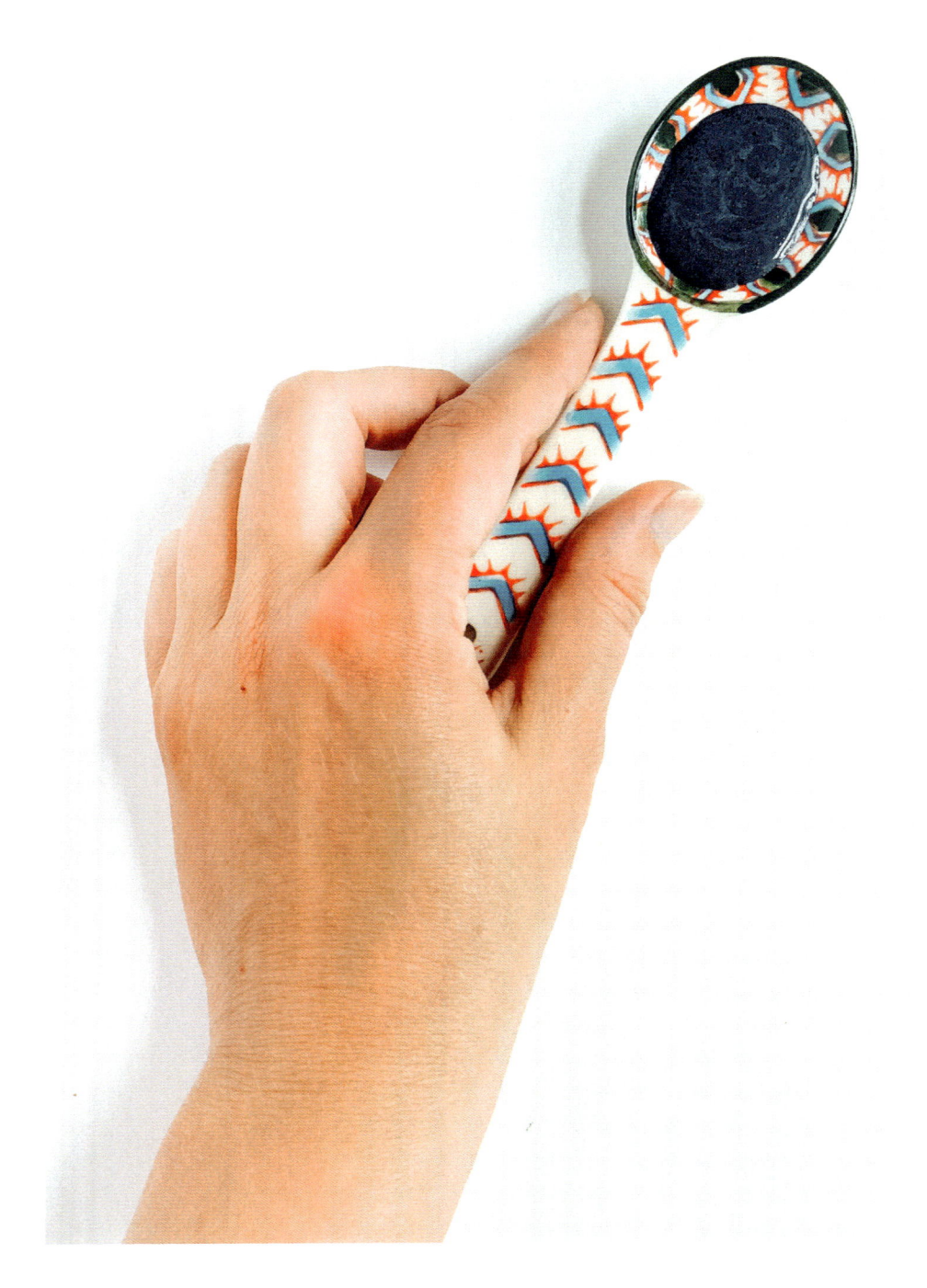

DIY CHARCOAL MASK

DIY FACE MASKS

*M*y charcoal face mask is easy to make and does an excellent job of deeply purifying your skin, leaving it cleansed and healthy. I've used all-natural ingredients: kaolin clay, jojoba oil, vegetable glycerin, rose hydrosol, lavender, tea tree, and rose geranium essential oils and of course activated charcoal!

This recipe is a copycat of a popular brand product. This recipe has all its goodness with similar natural ingredients, except its better, ha! It comes without the addition of any chemicals or preservatives. And also, let's not forget, it does not include the heavy price tag!

My homemade DIY face charcoal mask has a beautiful blue anthracite color and your skin will love it!

How to choose charcoal for your face mask?

Make sure it is food grade, 100% natural activated charcoal. The source can be from hardwood, coconut or bamboo.

PREP TIME: 10 MINUTES

TOTAL TIME: 10 MINUTES

MAKES: ONE APPLICATION

INGREDIENTS

- 6 teaspoons white kaolin clay
- 2 teaspoons activated charcoal powder
- 2 teaspoons rose flower water rose hydrosol
- 2 drops vegetable glycerin (optional)
- 1/4 teaspoon Jojoba oil (optional)
- 1 drop Lavender essential oil (optional)
- 1 drop Tea tree essential oil (optional)

INSTRUCTIONS

- Combine all ingredients together until it forms a liquid paste.
- Apply as an acne spot treatment for 15 minutes or on all your face (avoiding the eye and mouth area) for 5 minutes.
- Remove the homemade charcoal face mask with a warm wet cloth with a few drops of gentle soap (Castille soap) and massage your skin gently while doing so. Rinse your face gently with warm water and then finish with cold water to close your pores.
- Moisturize with rosehip oil or jojoba oil.
- Repeat once or twice a week.
- This clay mask recipe makes one application and can help clean the skin and reduce acne inflammation and redness.

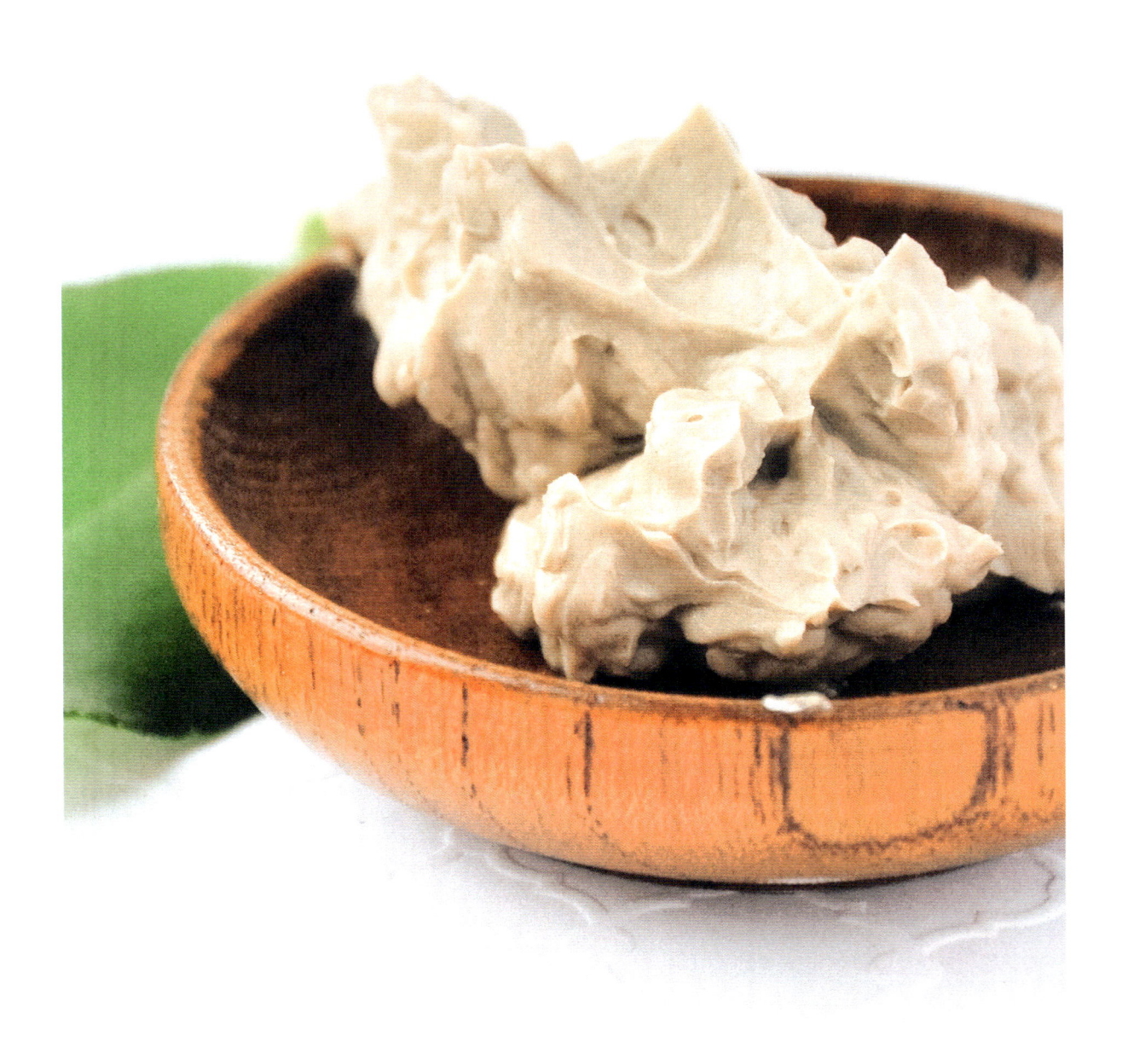

CLAY MASK FOR ACNE

DIY FACE MASKS

I love to use my bentonite clay mask recipe for acne as a spot treatment to reduce skin redness.

Due to its natural detoxification abilities, bentonite clay helps to treat skin inflammation. Acne can be caused by clogged pores, irregular skin cell shedding, bacterial overgrowth and excessive oil production – bentonite clay can help with all of these causes!

For best results, use this bentonite clay mask recipe for acne regularly. You may choose to do a detoxification protocol, in which you apply the mask for a few days in a row before applying once weekly as a part of your regular skincare routine. Over time, your pores will shrink, your skin's oil production will normalize and breakouts will clear up.

PREP TIME: 10 MINUTES

TOTAL TIME: 10 MINUTES

MAKES: ONE APPLICATION

INGREDIENTS

- 2 tablespoons of Bentonite clay
- 3 tablespoons of Chamomile flower water hydrosol
- 1 drops of Lavender essential oil
- 1 drops of Tea tree essential oil

INSTRUCTIONS

- Combine all ingredients together until it forms a thick paste
- Apply as a spot treatment for 15 minutes or on all your face (avoiding the eye area) for 5 minutes Remove the clay with a warm wet cloth and massage your skin gently while doing so.
- Rinse your face gently with warm water and then finish with cold water to close your pores.
- Moisturize with rosehip oil or jojoba oil.
- Repeat once a week.
- This clay mask recipe can help heal the skin and reduce inflammation and redness.

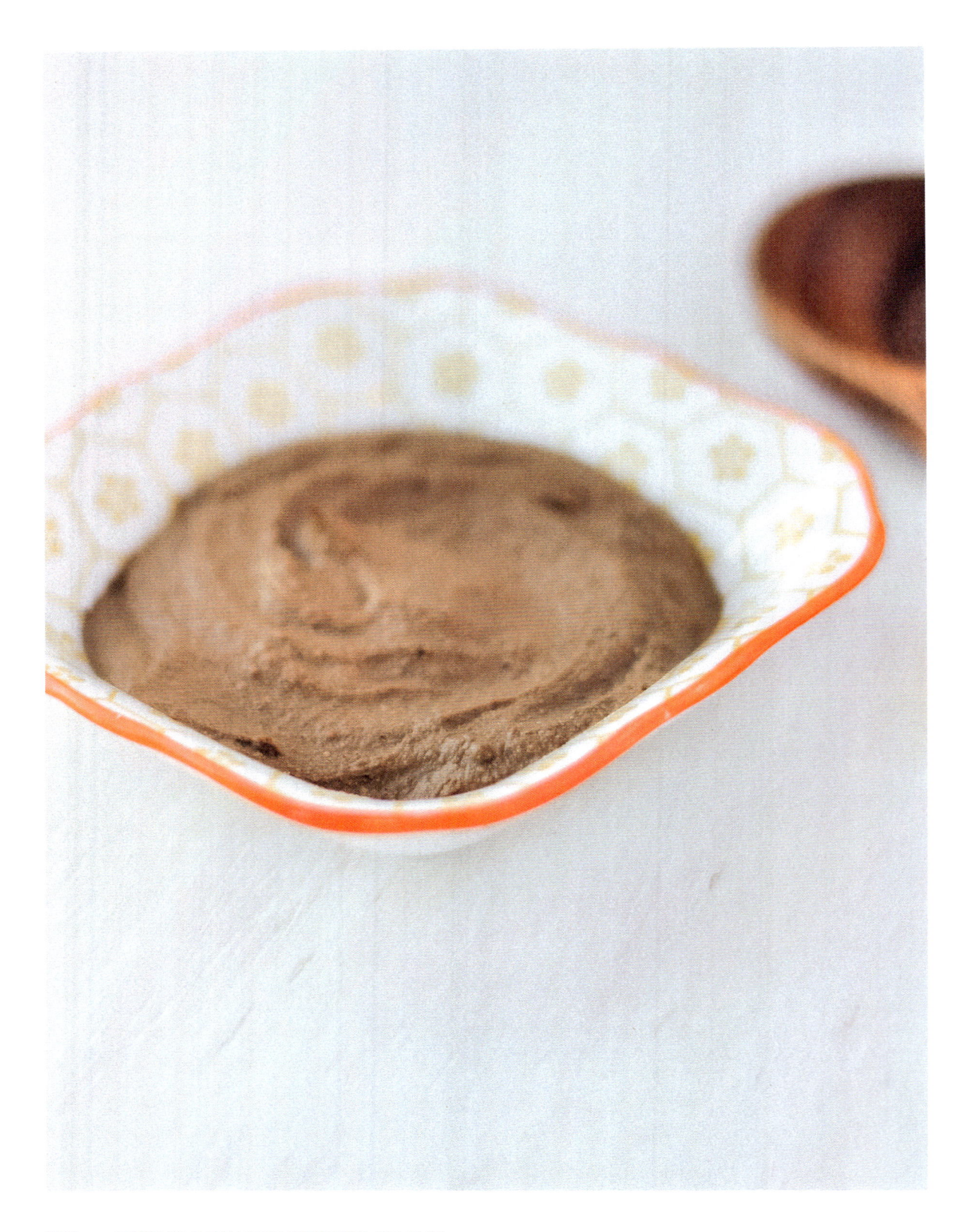

AYURVEDIC FACE MASK

DIY FACE MASKS

Ayurveda is an ancient system of life (ayur) knowledge (veda) originating from India thousands of years ago. In this Ayurvedic face mask recipe for acne, I have used sacred lotus seed powder, amla fruit powder, multani mitti clay powder and organic rose hydrosol.

PREP TIME: 10 MINUTES

TOTAL TIME: 10 MINUTES

MAKES: ONE APPLICATION

INGREDIENTS

- 1 teaspooon of sacred lotus seed powder (nelumbo nucifera seed powder)
- 1 teaspooon of amla fruit powder (emblica officinalis fruit powder)
- 1 teaspooon of multani mitti clay powder (fuller's earth clay)
- Organic Rose hydrosol or mineral water enough to form a thick paste.

INSTRUCTIONS

- Mix all the powders together in a glass, wood or ceramic bowl.
- Add the rose hydrosol or mineral water enough to form a thick paste.
- Do not use metal (spoon or bowl) as this can interfere with the clay properties.
- If you don't have a wooden or a plastic spoon, use your finger to mix the paste!
- Apply on your face for 15 mins or until the mask starts to become dry.
- Use every other day. You can also use this mask as a spot treatment daily before going to bed.

132   ORGANIC BEAUTY RECIPES BY EVE

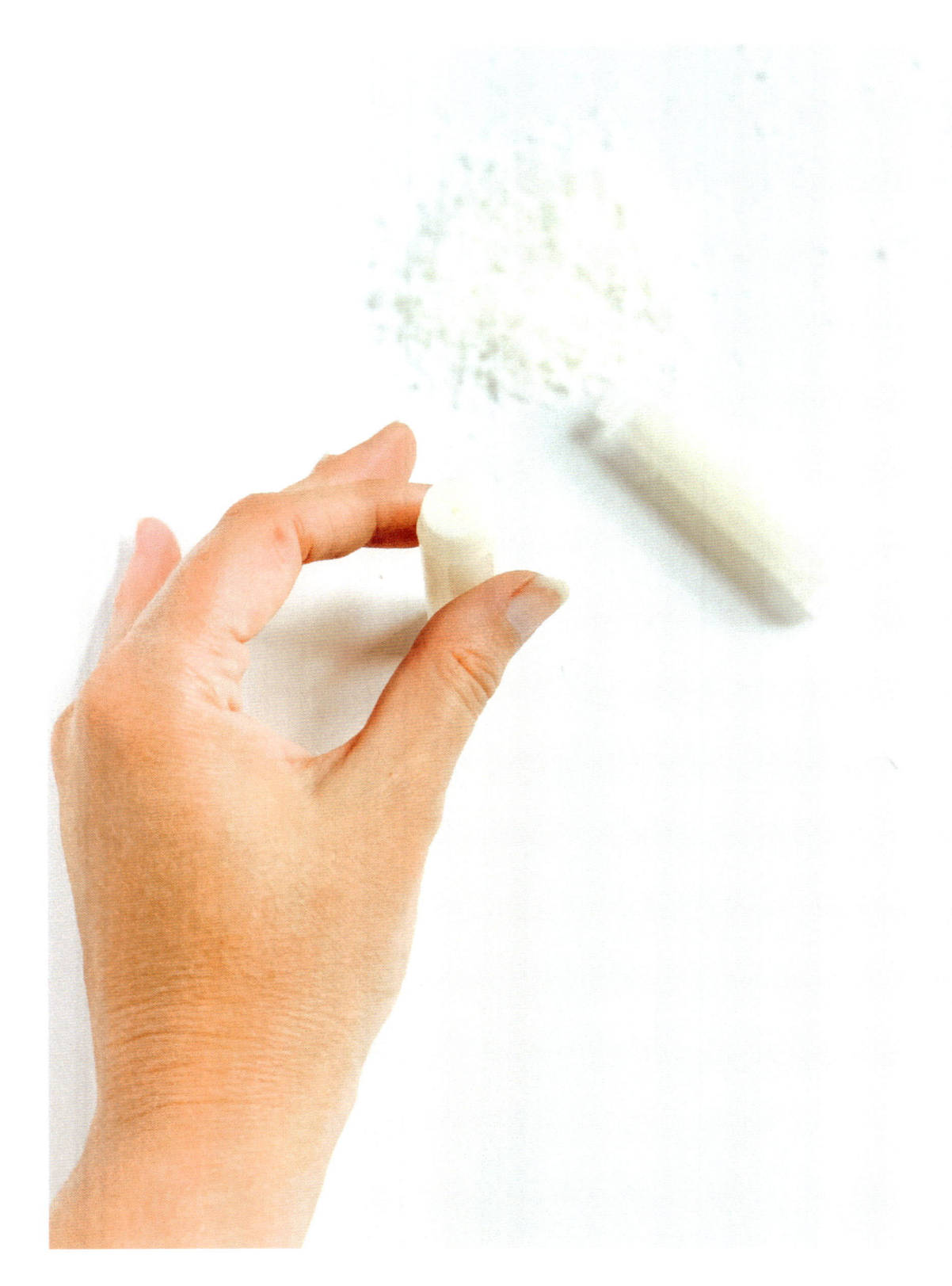

COCONUT OIL LIP BALM

LIP BALM RECIPES

For all the coco nuts out there, I've created this easy coconut oil lip balm recipe DIY, Step By Step recipe you can create right in your kitchen!

Coconut oil is excellent as a skin moisturiser and softener. I am also using castor oil to add extra shine but you could use liquid carrier oil like safflower oil or olive oil if you wanted something less shiny.

Beeswax is what will make your lip balm harden so don't skip this ingredient... Add some peppermint essential oil for a "fresh like" sensation!

If you choose refined coconut oil, it will not have the lovely coconut scent, opt in for the virgin non refined coconut oil; always organic please!

PREP TIME: 10 MINUTES

COOK TIME: 5 MINUTES

TOTAL TIME: 15 MINUTES

MAKES: 8 LIP BALM

INGREDIENTS

- 2 tablespoons of organic beeswax
- 4 tablespoons of organic virgin non refined coconut oil
- 2 tablespoons organic castor oil
- 15 drops of organic peppermint essential oil
- 8 plastic lip balm containers

INSTRUCTIONS

- Gather all the ingredients and add the beeswax, castor oil and coconut oil in a double boiler or a pan filled with water on low to medium heat.
- Once melted, add the essential oil if desired and mix well.
- Pour the liquid wax immediately in the lip balm containers and fill them to the top. If it has already starting to harden, don't panic! Put it back into the double boiler for a few seconds until it melts again and pour the rest of the liquid wax in the lip balm containers.
- Wait one hour or two until the wax starts to harden then you can use the lip balm right away!
- If it is a hot day, you can pop the lip balm containers in the fridge so the lip balm hardens more quickly.

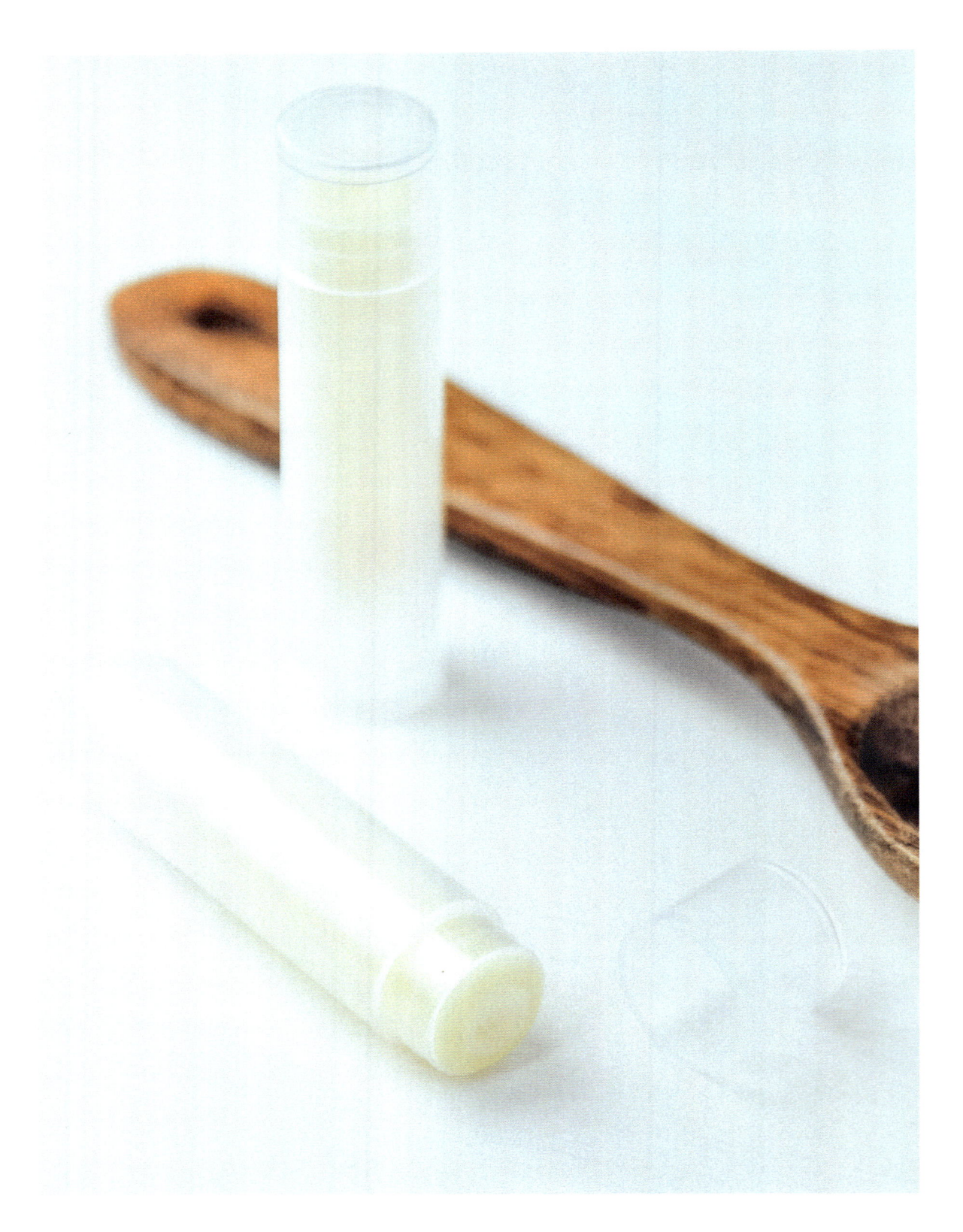

HONEY LIP BALM

LIP BALM RECIPES

*M*aking this honey lip balm recipe has saved me from dry and chapped lips during winter. Honey is antibacterial, antifungal, and antiseptic which helps moisturize chapped lips and promotes healing. Truly a miracle of nature for your lips!

This honey lip balm recipe requires few ingredients and it very easy to make at home. In this recipe, I use coconut oil, sunflower oil, beeswax and of course honey. I recommend using a liquid organic honey as it will be easier to mix with the oils and beeswax than a creamed honey.

PREP TIME: 10 MINUTES

COOK TIME: 5 MINUTES

TOTAL TIME: 15 MINUTES

MAKES: 7 LIP BALMS

INGREDIENTS

- 4 teaspoons of organic beeswax pellets
- 3 teaspoons of organic coconut oil
- 1 teaspoon of raw organic liquid honey
- 3 teaspoons of organic sunflower seed oil
- 5 drops of peppermint essential oil.
- 7 lip balm containers

INSTRUCTIONS

- Melt beeswax, oils, and honey in a double boiler on low to medium heat. If you do not have a double boiler, simply use an aluminum bowl placed in a pan filled with warm water.
- Once the beeswax has melted, take it off the heat and start whipping with an electric or manual mixer until the liquid becomes frosty and the honey well blended. (At first, you will see the honey at the bottom of the oils, which means you need to mix more!).
- If the wax has already starting to harden, don't panic! Put it back into the double boiler for a few seconds until it melts again and pour the rest the containers.
- Let it cool for 2 hours until it has completely solidified.
- Apply on your lips as often as needed!
- The shelf life of this honey lip balm is about 1 year, depending on the shelf life of the oils and you have used. It does not need to be refrigerated.

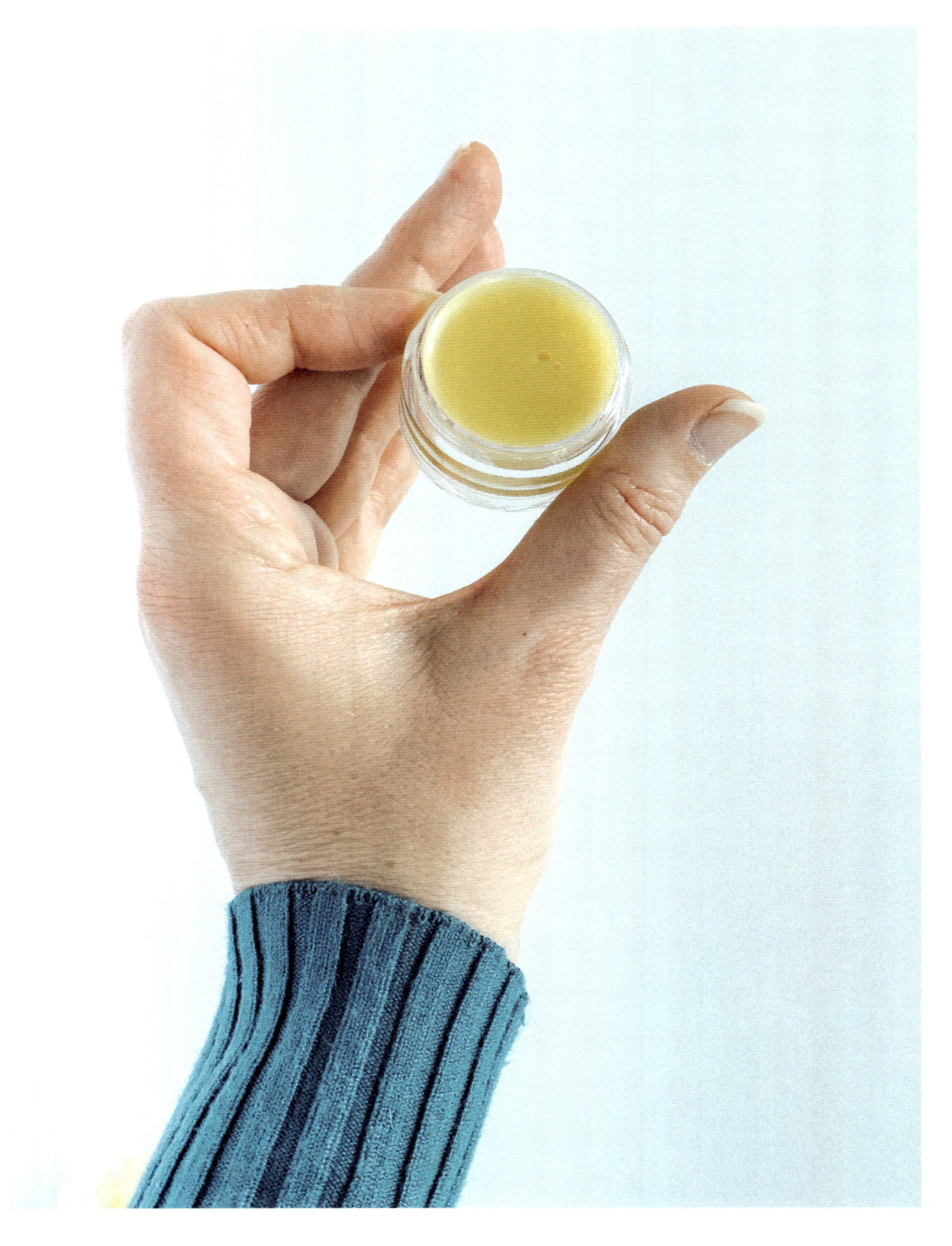

VEGAN LIP BALM WITHOUT BEESWAX

LIP BALM RECIPES

Are you Vegan or concerned to use beeswax because of the impact on the environment? Here is my DIY lip balm recipe with Candelilla Wax which will keep your lips soft and plump while having less impact on our friends the bees!

Vegan lip balms can be hard to find or expensive, which is why making your own lip balm is the best thing to do. This DIY lip balm recipe is without beeswax, 100% vegan and cruelty-free.

PREP TIME: 5 MINUTES

COOKING TIME: 10 MINUTES

TOTAL TIME: 15 MINUTES

MAKES: 6 LIPS BALMS

INGREDIENTS

- 1 teaspoon of Candelilla wax or Carnauba Wax
- 4 teaspoons of Olive Oil
- 2 teaspoons of Castor Oil
- 2 teaspoons of Cocoa Butter
- 15 drops spearmint essential oil
- 6 lip balm containers

INSTRUCTIONS

- Add the proper amounts of carnauba wax or candelilla wax and cocoa butter to a double boiler.
- Melt your candelilla wax and cocoa butter in a double boiler.
- Add olive oil, castor oil to the boiler and allow melting thoroughly on low heat. Do not overheat!
- Add essential oils (optional) and mix well.
- Pour your mixture into lip balm tubes and allow cooling for 2 hours until it has solidified.

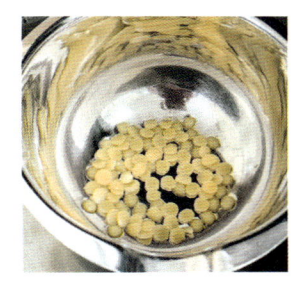

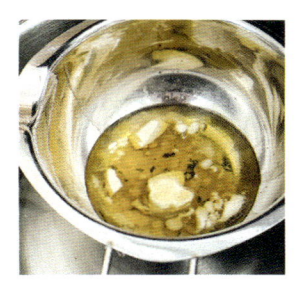

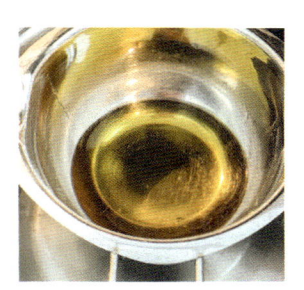

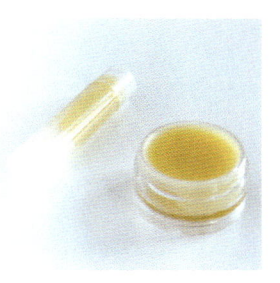

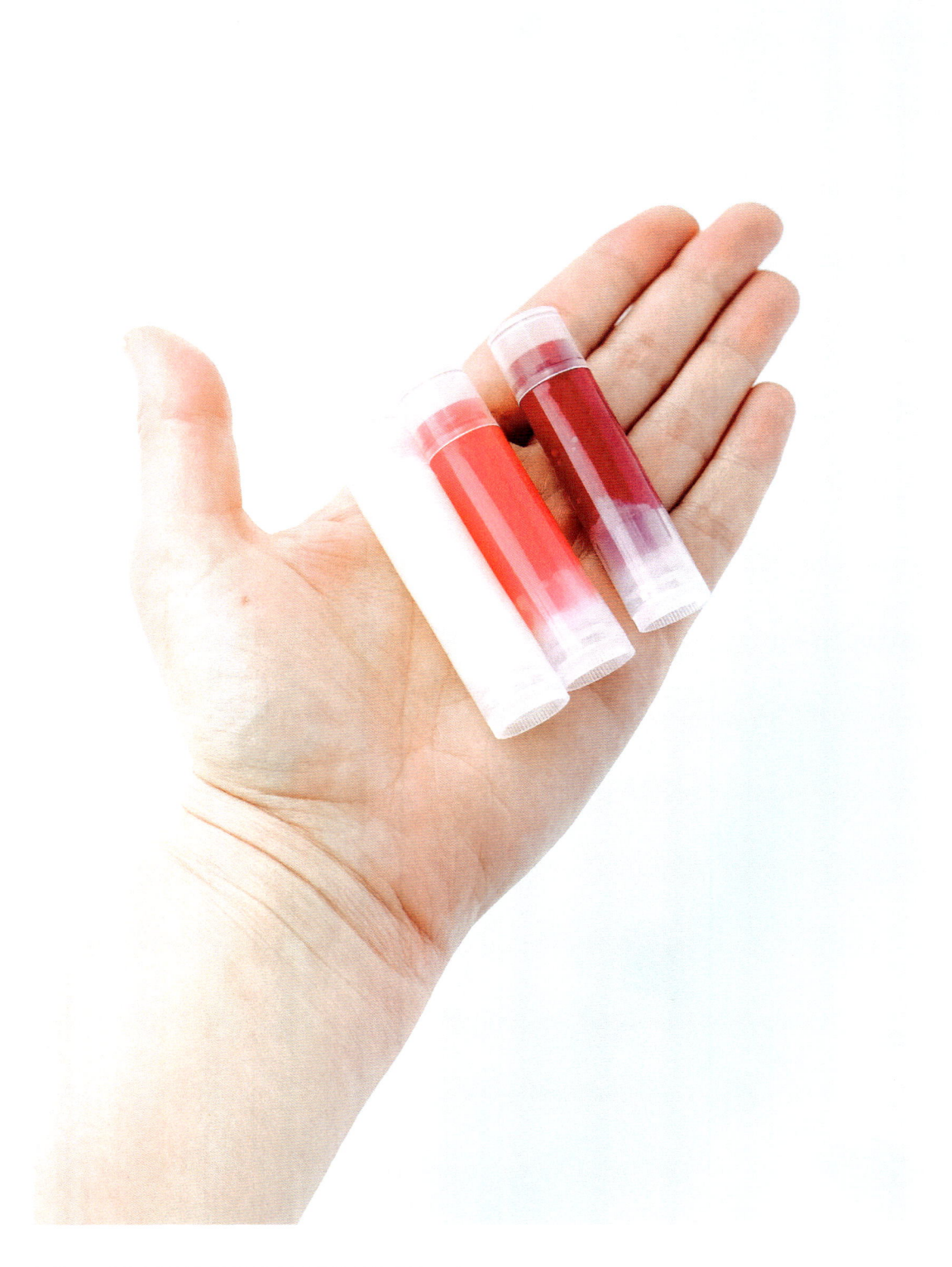

TINTED LIP BALM WITH COCONUT OIL AND SOYWAX

LIP BALM RECIPES

If you wonder if you can make tinted coconut lip balm without beeswax and how to make a vegan lip balm, you've come to the right place! My all-natural vegan lip balm recipe with coconut oil and soy wax will make your lips plush and smooth.

You will find also different DIY tinted lip balm options if you are feeling adventurous which includes a different shade of pink to red...

Customizing your lip balm color to your liking is half the fun!

PREP TIME: 5 MINUTES

COOK TIME: 5 MINUTES

TOTAL TIME: 10 MINUTES

MAKES: 2 LIP BALMS

INGREDIENTS

- 3 teaspoons of organic coconut oil
- 2 teaspoons of soywax
- 4 drops peppermint or rosemary essential oil OPTIONAL
- 1 pinch beetroot powder or micas OPTIONAL
- 3 drops natural vegetable colorants (adjust more or less depending on the intensity desired) OPTIONAL

INSTRUCTIONS

- Melt the raw coconut oil and soy wax over low heat in a small stainless steel or glass bowl, or using a double boiler, and stir until melted.
- Once melted, add the essential oil if desired and mix well.
- Remove the bowl from heat and your desired colorant if you wish.
- Pour the mixture into lip balm tubes and set aside for one hour to set.
- You can keep it at room temperature for up to 6 months.

Tip **YOU CAN ADJUST THE SOFTNESS** of the lip balm by removing 1/2 teaspooons of soywax. If you want this lip balm harder, then add 1/2 teaspooons of soywax!

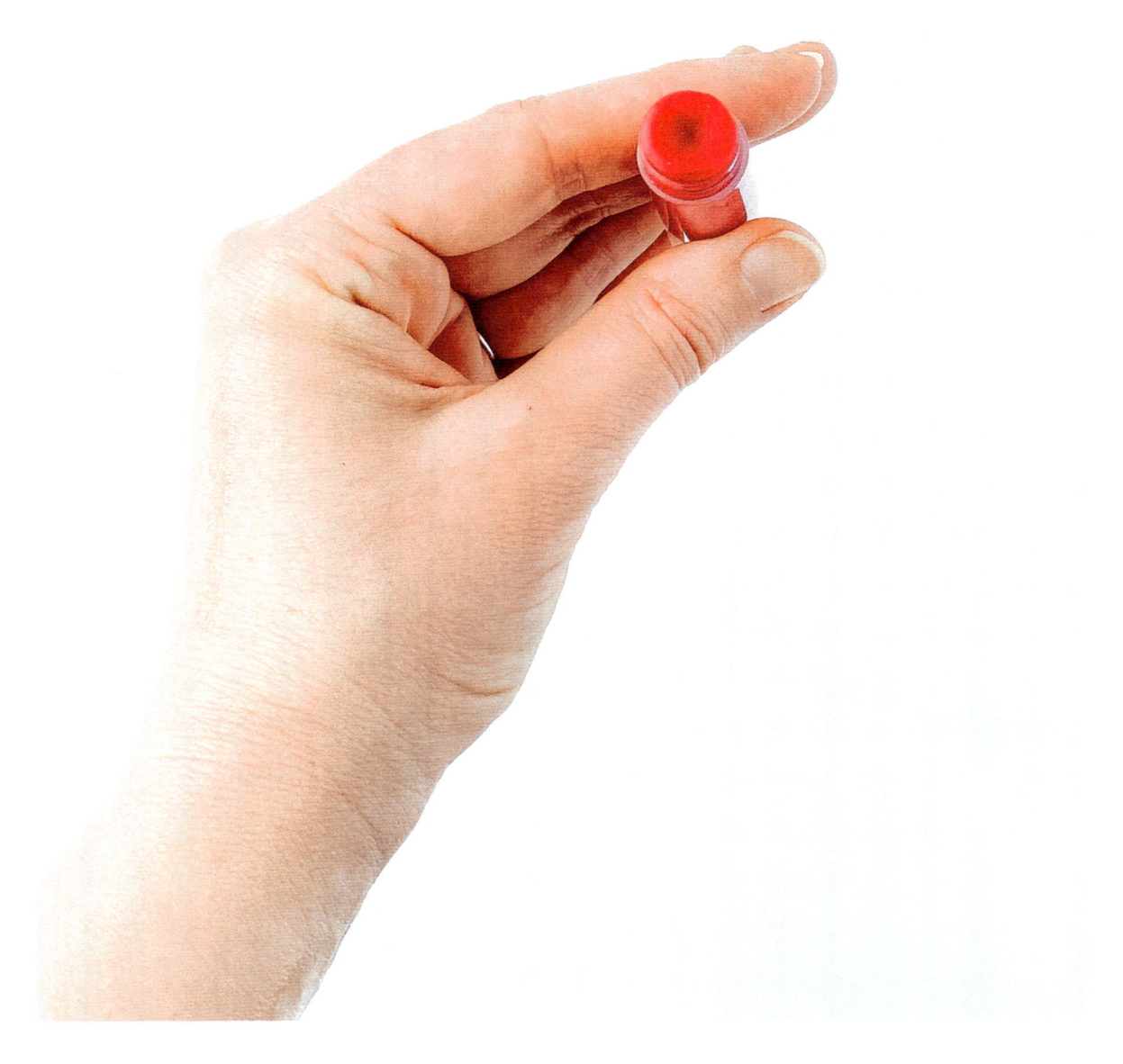

HOW TO TINT YOUR DIY LIP BALM NATURALLY?

LIP BALM RECIPES

Add a hint of beautiful sheen and color to your lips by incorporating beetroot powder, micas or vegetable and natural colorants in your natural tinted lip balm recipe.

Beetroot Powder give a natural pink to red pigmentation on lips.

Mica pigments are natural minerals that are purified and then crushed, and range from matte to sparkling or opalescent. This powder is considered safe for lips, eyes, and cheeks.

Grenadine Natural vegetable colorant found on Aroma zone. This 100% vegetable dye-based on organic vegetable oils allows you to color your lip balm and lipstick in pink to light red tones. Love the bright pink color!

Natural colorant red kiss found on aroma zone with carmine. This natural carmine concentrated on oily support is ideal for the formulation of lipsticks and gloss. It brings an intense red coloring with excellent hold. Please note this is NOT vegan!

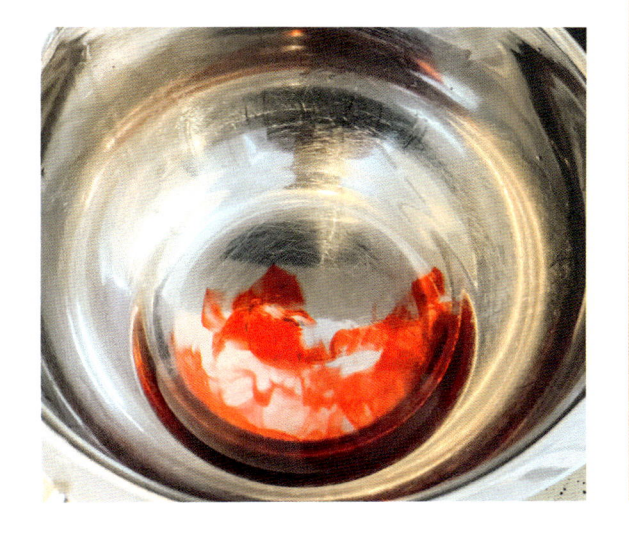

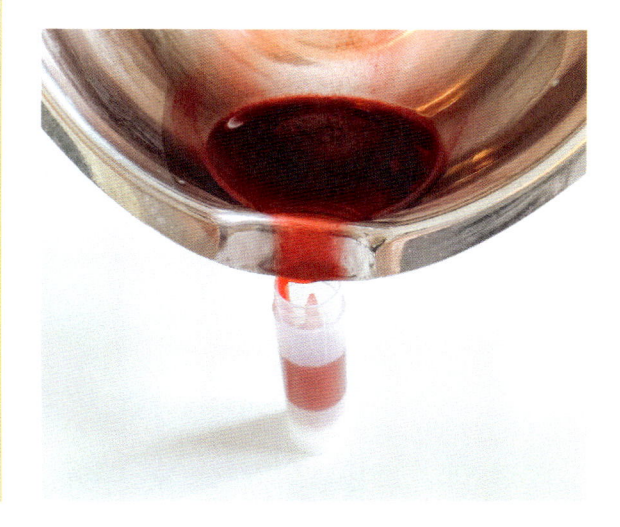

142   ORGANIC BEAUTY RECIPES BY EVE

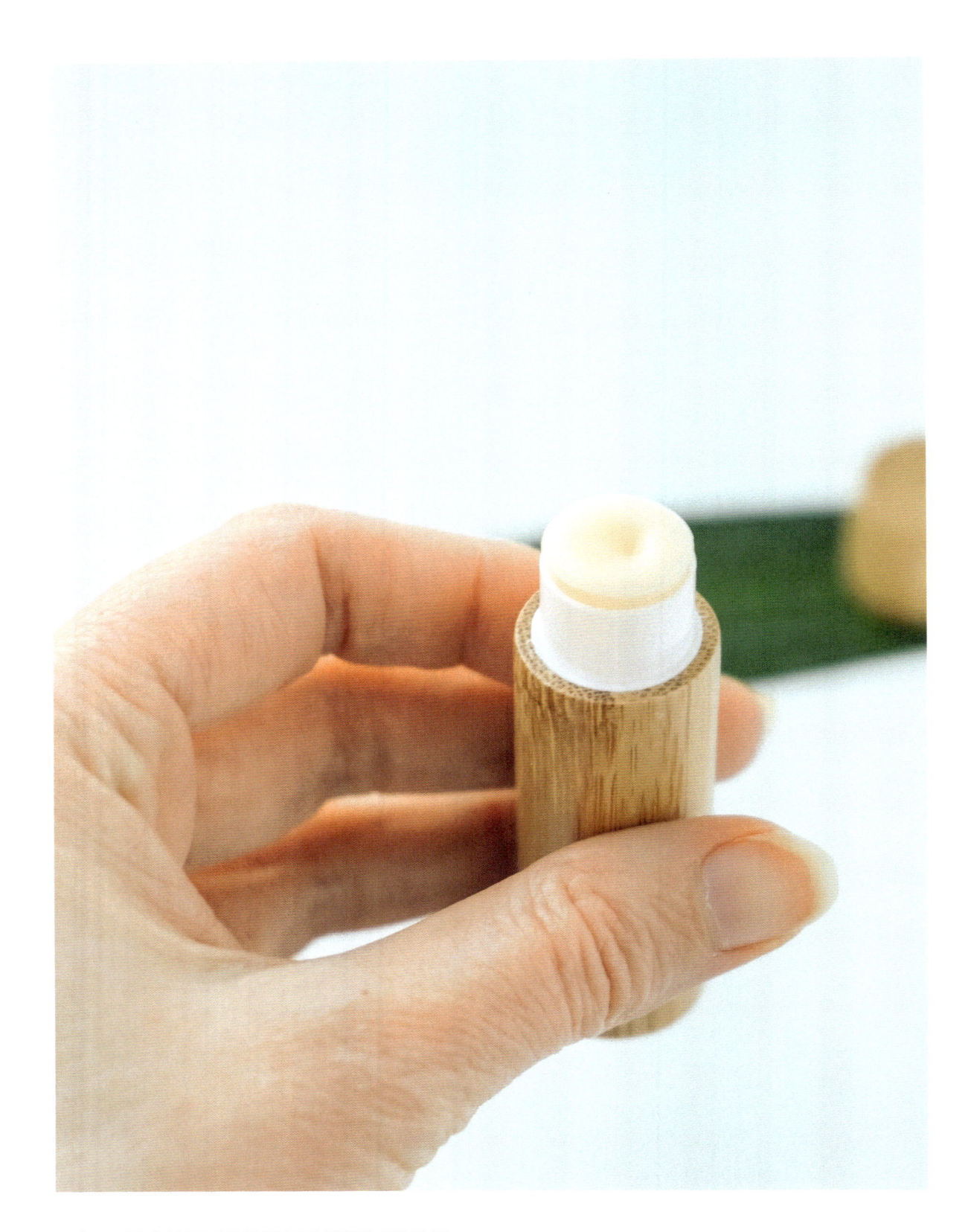

HOMEMADE PEPPERMINT LIP BALM

LIP BALM RECIPES

To provide optimum care and extra nourishment for your lips, try on my DIY recipe of homemade lip balm with peppermint. I've created a copycat of a famous brand name peppermint lip balm with beeswax, avocado oil, jojoba oil, hemp seed oil and of course peppermint essential oil.

PREP TIME: 5 MINUTES

COOK TIME: 5 MINUTES

TOTAL TIME: 10 MINUTES

MAKES: 8 LIP BALMS

INGREDIENTS

- 4 teaspoons of organic beeswax pellets
- 3 teaspoons of organic avocado oil
- 2 teaspoons of organic hemp seed oil
- 2 teaspoons of jojoba oil
- 10 drops peppermint essential oil
- 8 lip balm containers

INSTRUCTIONS

- Melt beeswax, oils in a double boiler on low to medium heat. If you do not have a double boiler, simply use an aluminum bowl placed in a pan filled with warm water.
- Once melted, add the peppermint essential oil. Mix well.
- Pour immediately into the lip balm containers.
- If it has already starting to harden, don't panic! Put it back into the double boiler for a few seconds until it melts again and pour the rest the containers.
- Let it cool for 2 hours until it has completely solidified.
- Apply on your lips as often as needed!
- The shelf life of this peppermint lip balm is about 1 year, depending on the shelf life of the oils and you have used. It does not need to be refrigerated.

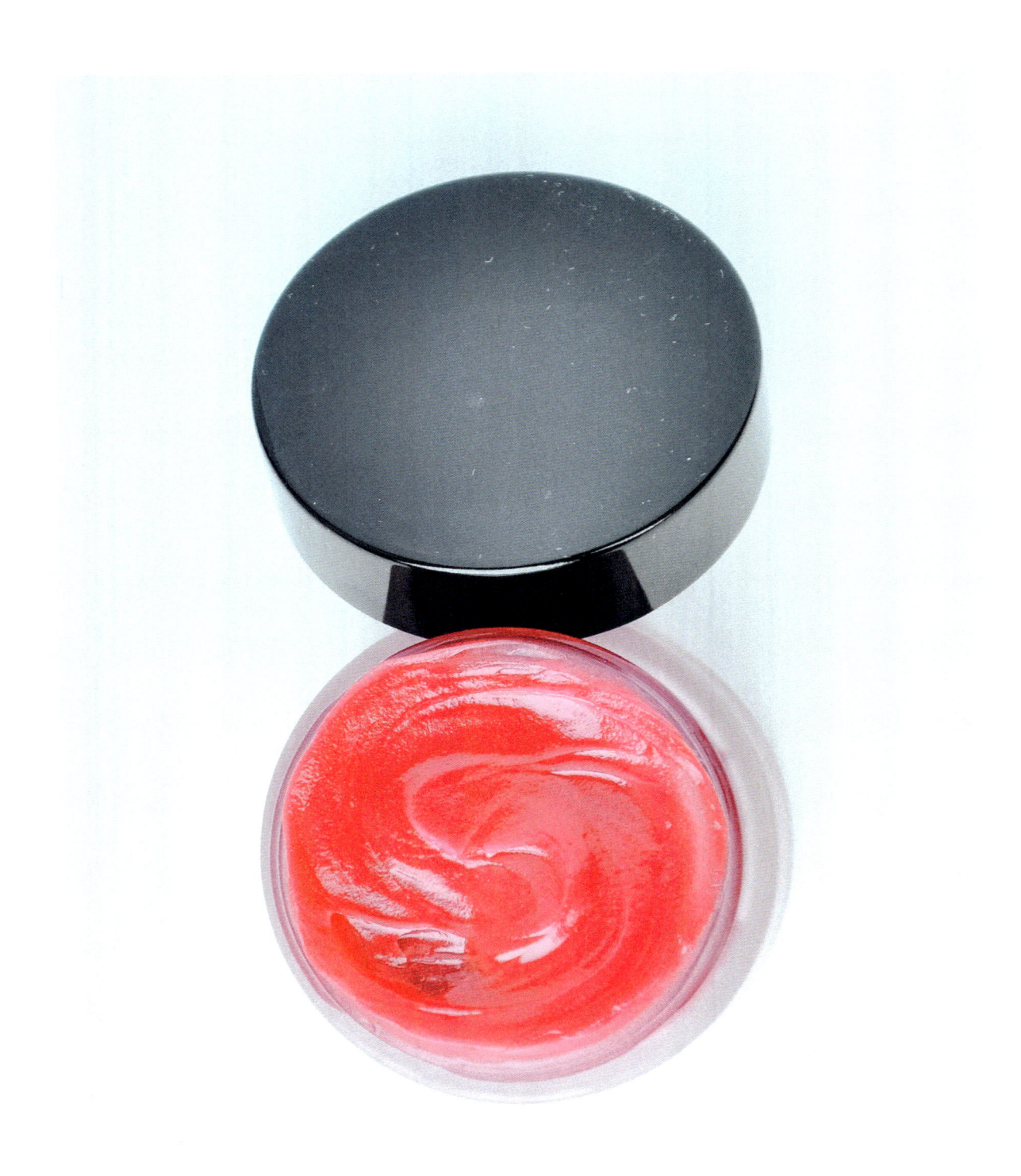

HOW TO MAKE PINK LIP GLOSS WITH BEETROOT

LIP GLOSS RECIPES

*This pink lip gloss recipe with beetroot provides a light, shiny texture and a bright pink pop of color. I've used white beeswax, shea butter, coconut oil, sunflower oil and peppermint essential oil.

PREP TIME: 5 MINUTES

COOK TIME: 5 MINUTES

TOTAL TIME: 10 MINUTES

MAKES: 8 LIP BALMS

INGREDIENTS

- 1 teaspoon of white organic beeswax
- 2 teaspoons of organic shea butter
- 3 teaspoons of organic castor oil
- 1 teaspoon of organic sunflower oil
- 1 teaspoon of coconut oil
- 1 teaspoon of organic beetroot powder OR 1/2 teaspoon organic beetroot juice concentrate
- 5 drops of peppermint essential oil optional
- 3 drops Grapefruit seed extract to help with preservation
- 8 lip balm containers

INSTRUCTIONS

- Melt the Shea butter, castor oil, sunflower oil, coconut oil and beeswax together in a double boiler or an aluminum bowl inside a pan filled with warm water on low to medium heat.
- Once melted, take the aluminum bowl outside the heat with gloves so you don't burn yourself.
- If you are using the beetroot powder, make sure the powder is very fine or else you will end up with a grainy lip gloss. Blend the beetroot powder in a fast blender until it is a very fine powder.
- Add the teaspoon of beetroot powder OR 1/2 teaspoon of beetroot juice concentrate.
- Add the essential oil if desired and the grapeseed extract for preservation.
- Mix well for a few minutes with a spoon until the beetroot is completely dissolved.
- The mixture should look like a thick lip gloss, very glossy and easy to apply to the lips.

If your lip gloss is too liquid and stays more like oil, add the aluminum bowl into another bowl of cold water so it cools down the ingredients.

This recipe can last up to 2 months or longer if you add the grapeseed extract.

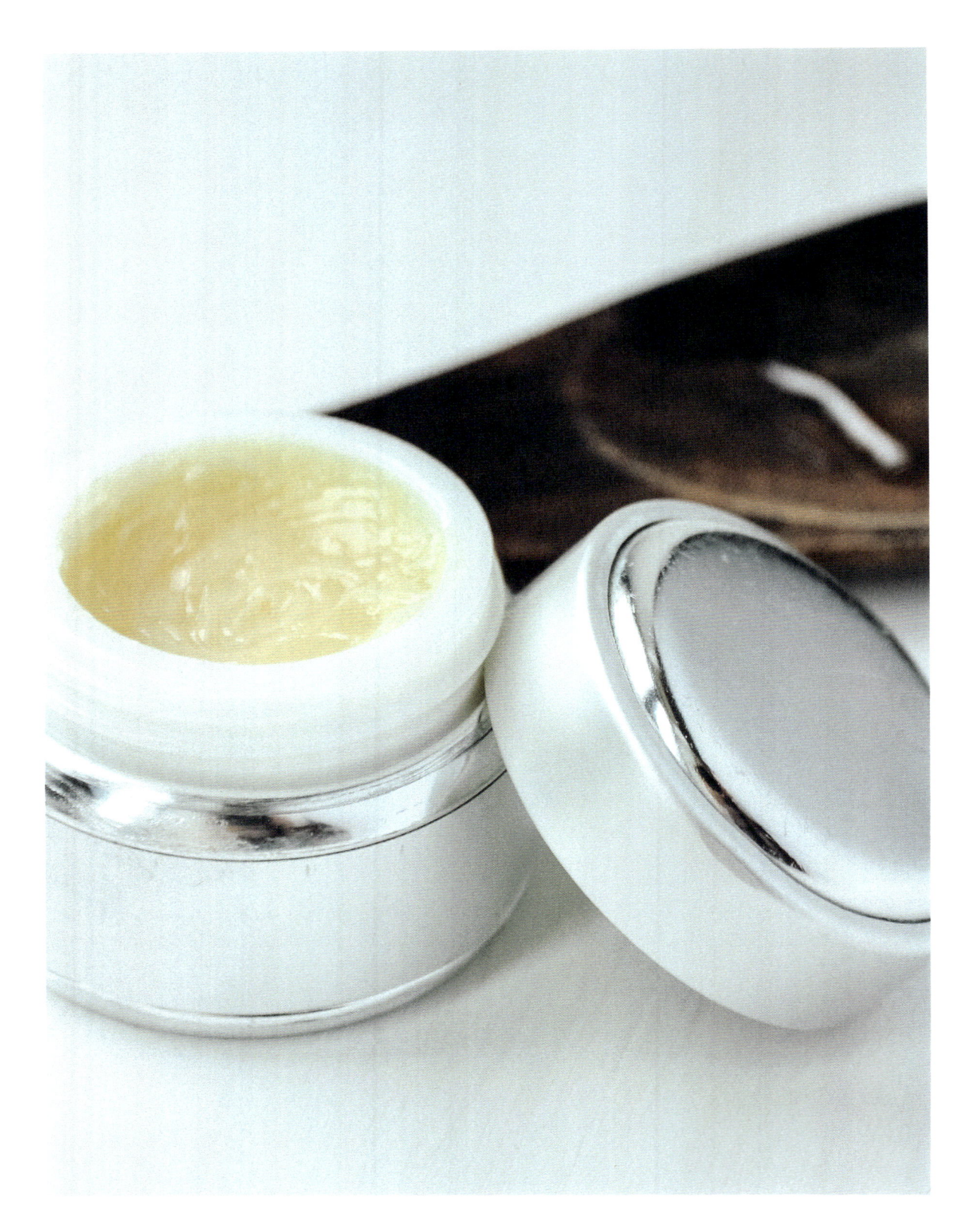

HONEY LIP GLOSS

LIP GLOSS RECIPES

*T*his honey lip gloss recipe has only 4 ingredients, organic liquid honey, cocoa butter, castor oil, and beeswax. It is a clear and thick lip gloss recipe great repair for damaged, dry or chapped lips.

This homemade 100% natural recipe takes advantage of the natural shine, sweet taste and healing properties of the honey. It's a fun easy to make lip gloss recipe to add to your DIY beauty arsenal.

You can follow the step by step tutorial below if this is your first time making lip gloss.

PREP TIME: 10 MINUTES

COOK TIME: 5 MINUTES

TOTAL TIME: 15 MINUTES

MAKES: 1 OZ

INGREDIENTS

- 1 teaspoon organic beeswax
- 2 teaspoons organic cocoa butter non-refined
- 4 teaspoon organic castor oil
- 1 teaspoon of organic liquid honey
- Essential oils optional
- 5 drops of peppermint essential oil

INSTRUCTIONS

- Melt the cocoa butter, castor oil, and beeswax together in a double boiler or an aluminum bowl inside a pan filled with warm water on low to medium heat.
- Once melted add the liquid honey.
- Mix well with a whip until it is foamy for a few minutes.
- Add the essential oils if desired.
- Mix well for a few seconds.
- Take off the heat and pour immediately into a 1 oz nice container.
- Let cool for 1 hour and the lip balm will solidify.
- This recipe can last up to 6 months (depending on the shelf life of the oil and butter you use)
- Use on your lips as needed!

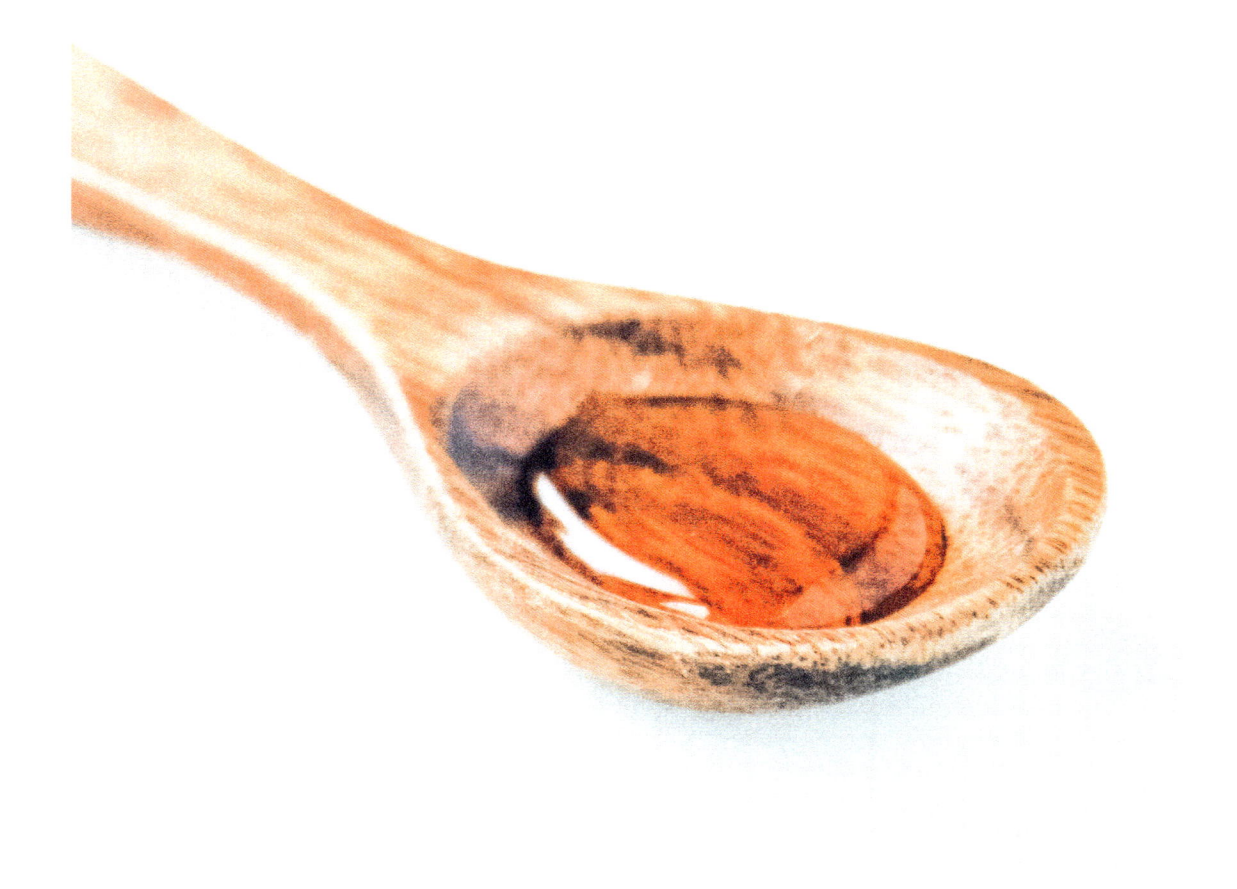

TUTORIAL DIY HONEY LIP GLOSS

LIP GLOSS RECIPES

Step 1
Melt the cocoa butter, castor oil, and beeswax together in a double boiler or an aluminum bowl inside a pan filled with warm water on low to medium heat.

Step 2
Once melted add the liquid honey and mix well for a few minutes until it is foamy with a whip. You want the honey well blended with the wax, butter, and oil. You don't want to have the honey at the bottom of the bowl or it will separate later.

Step 3
Add the essential oils if desired. Mix well for a few seconds.

Step 4
Take the bowl off the heat (make sure you use heat proof gloves not to burn yourself) and pour immediately into a 1 oz nice container before it starts to solidify.

Step 5
Let cool for 1 hour and the honey lip gloss will solidify but will be soft enough to be applied with your (clean and dry) finger on your lips.

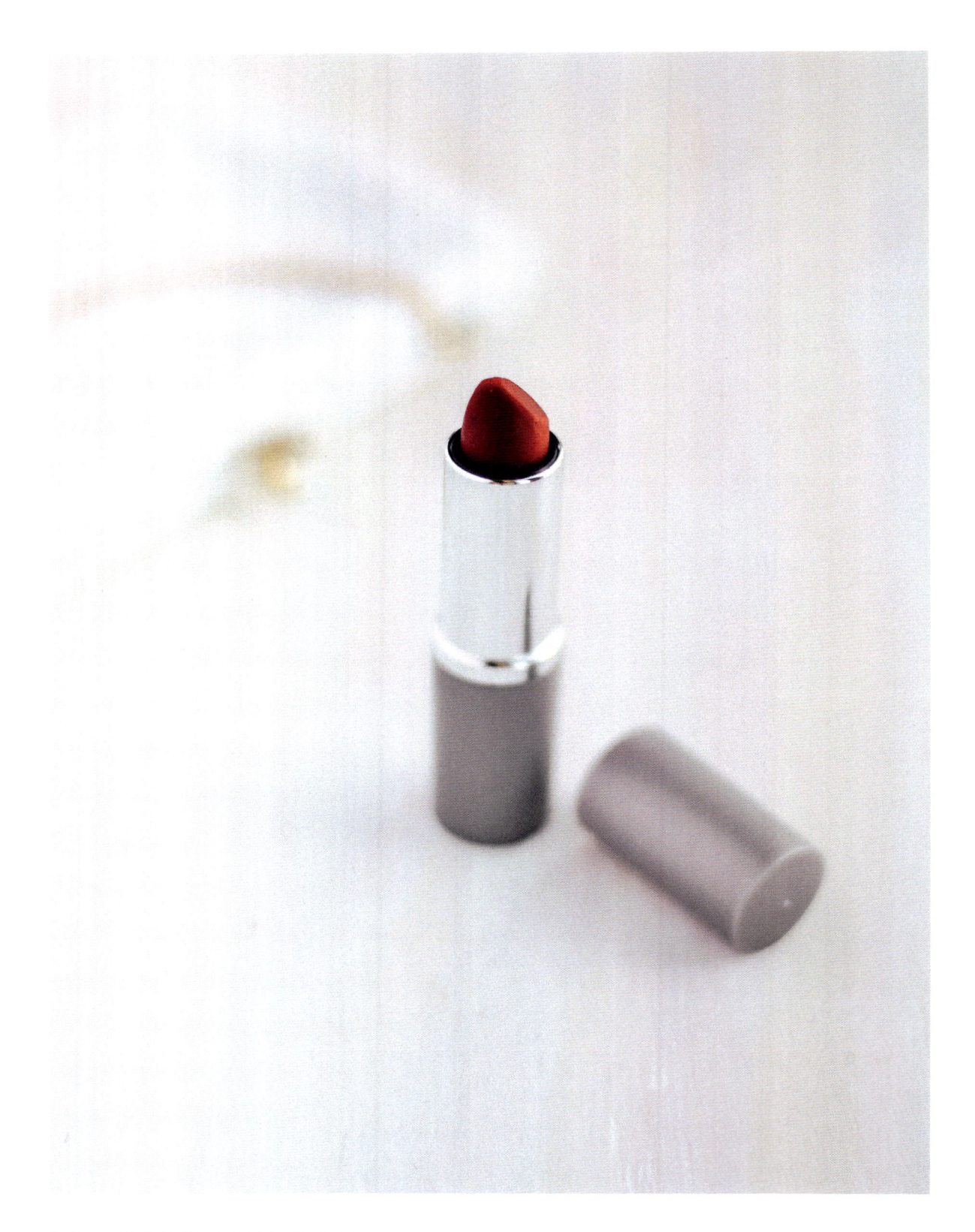

HOW TO MAKE LIPSTICK LIKE A PRO

LIPSTICK RECIPES

I wanted to make a homemade lipstick that looks like the one you get in stores. Turns out it is not as hard as you can imagine. Packaging like this high-grade lipstick tube and a few tools can make a world of difference in your product finish!

Lipsticks really do have the ability to add that magic touch to a woman's appearance that makes you feel like you can conquer the world.

If you're worried about all the toxic chemicals used in commercially produced lipsticks (and you should be!), it's time to make the shift to natural, homemade lipsticks.

PREP TIME: 30 MINUTES

COOK TIME: 5 MINUTES

TOTAL TIME: 35 MINUTES

MAKES: 4 LIPSTICKS

INGREDIENTS

- 1 teaspoon natural red colorant 10% Natural carmine CI 75470 (obtained from cochineal in a sunflower oil carrier)
- 1 teaspoon rice wax 10%
- 1 teaspoon carnauba wax 10%
- 1 teaspoon candelila wax 10%
- 3 teaspoons organic refined shea butter 30%
- 2 teaspoons organic castor oil 20%
- 1 teaspoon organic camellia seed oil 10%
- You'll need silicon mold for lipstick you can get this one from Aroma Zone (French company so keep in mind you will have to pay import custom fees if you don't live in France.) or you can find one on amazon.com
- Lipstick tubes– If using an old lipstick container one make sure it is clean, dried and sterilized.

INSTRUCTIONS

- Melt the oil, butter and waxes in a double boiler on low heat until melted.
- Add the colorant, mix well.
- Pour in the empty lipstick tube as explained in the tutorial.
- Put in the freezer for 15 minutes.
- Unmold as per instructions below.
- Use within one year.

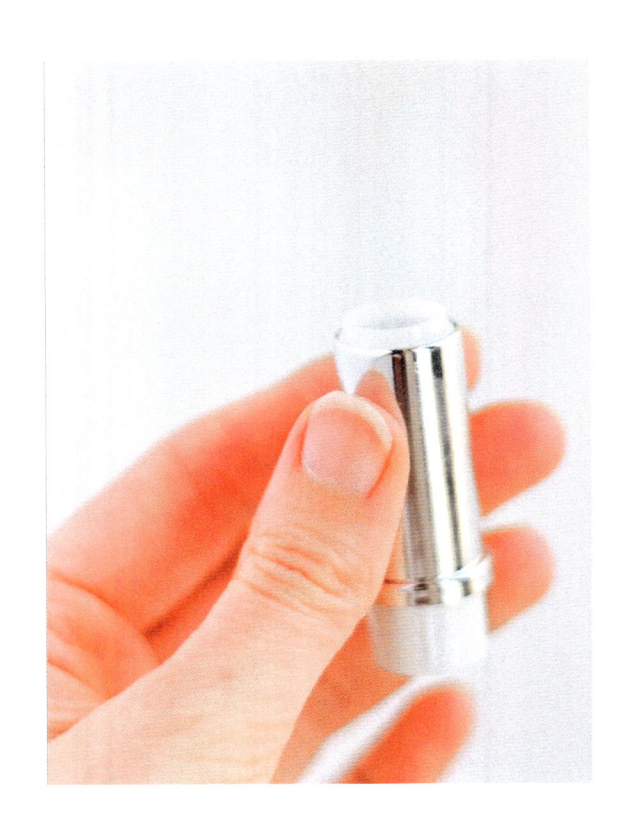

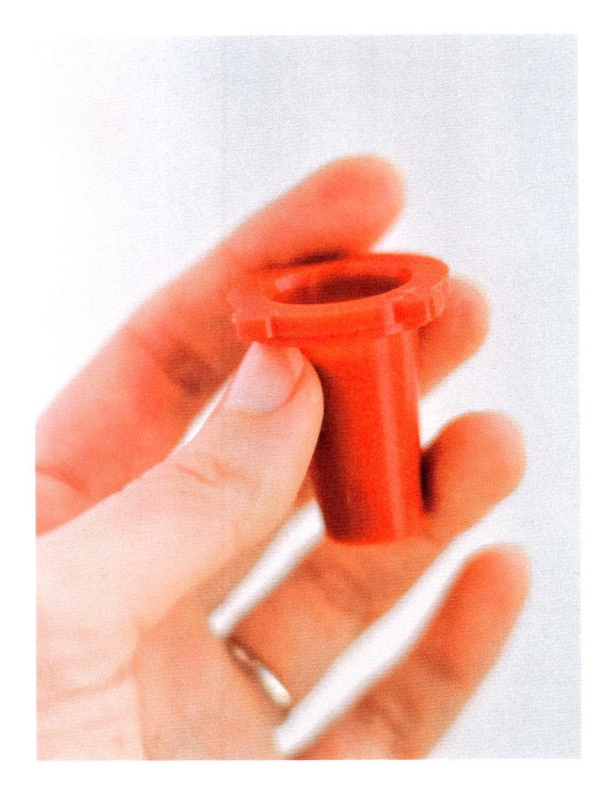

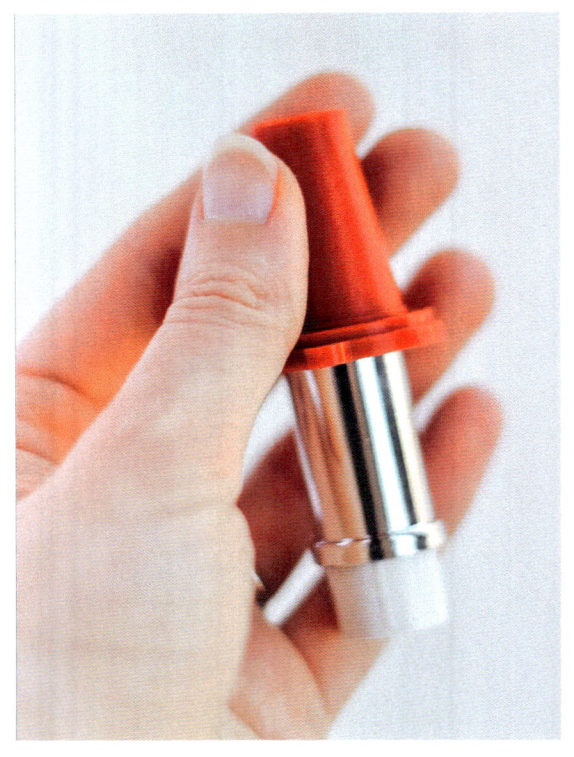

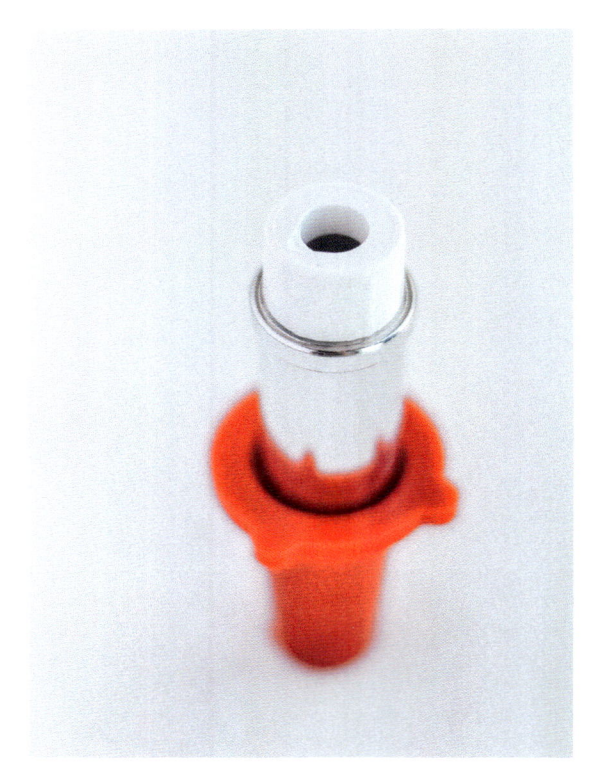

152   ORGANIC BEAUTY RECIPES BY EVE

TUTORIAL HOW TO USE THE LIPSTICK SILICON MOLD

LIPSTICK RECIPES

Step 1
Remove the cover and the base of the lipstick container.

Step 2
Turn the bottom white part of the mechanism to the maximum in order to have the transparent inner part up.

Step 3
Clip the transparent inner part in the lipstick mold.

Step 4
Put the lipstick mold upside down on a table and start pouring through the bottom of the body of the empty case.

Step 5
Pour the melted lipstick mixture quickly inside the lipstick container. Do not to exceed the little white gate!

Step 6
Place the entire (+ mold body of the case) 15 minutes in the freezer in the same position as casting.

Step 7
To unmold, put the lipstick upright and unmold very gently the silicone mold.

Step 8
Turn the mechanism to retract the lipstick stick inside the body of the container, then put the base and the cover on.

Step 9
Clean the silicone mold with warm water and soap. Let dry before you use it again. Voila, you are done!

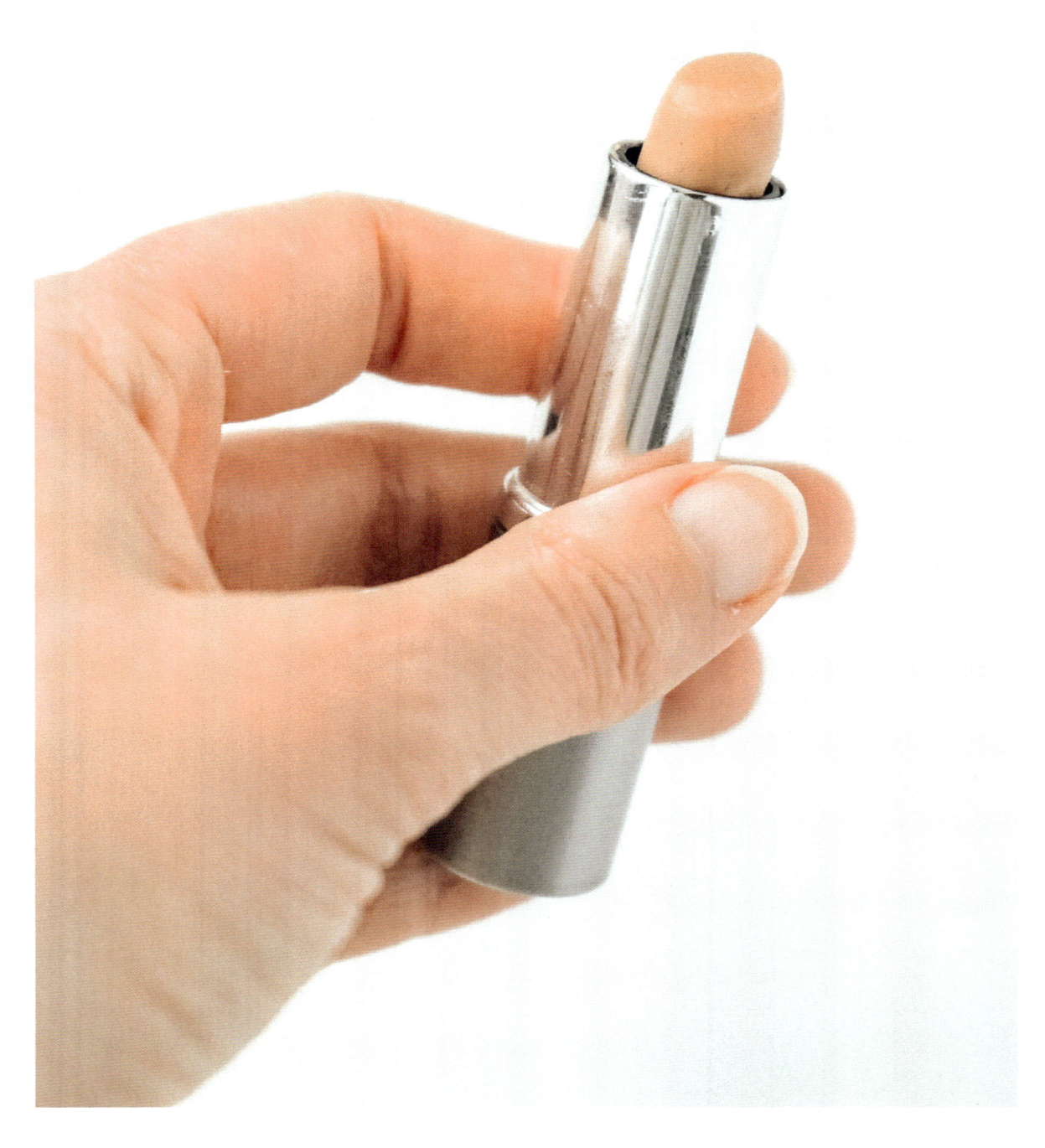

DIY MATTE LIPSTICK WITHOUT BEESWAX

LIPSTICK RECIPES

After a lot of trial and error, I created this amazing vegan DIY matte lipstick which will surely become your makeup staple. This homemade lipstick has a nude color with a matte effect. This is achieved with the use of zinc oxide and rice flour. My matte lipstick recipe is a base that can be customized to your liking. It is vegan since I do not use beeswax.

This recipe is a little advanced because of the use of the mold, which can be tricky. It does also require more ingredients than my usual DIY recipes. So please ensure you have made a lip balm recipe before tackling this lipstick recipe!

PREP TIME: 10 MINUTES

COOK TIME: 15 MINUTES

TOTAL TIME: 25 MINUTES

MAKES: 3 LIPSTICKS

INGREDIENTS

- 1/4 teaspoon honey beige or bronze mica Try to get mica that is not too shimmery to accentuate the matte lipstick effect.
- 1/4 teaspoon zync oxyde
- 1/2 teaspoon rice flour (oriza sativa flour)
- 1/2 teaspoon camelia seed oil
- 1 teaspoon rice bran wax
- 1 teaspoon Carnauba wax
- 1 teaspoon candelilla wax
- 5 teaspoons refine shea butter
- 7 teaspoons sunflower oil or jojoba oil or camelia seed oil
- 1 silicon mold for lipstick you can get this one from Aroma Zone or on amazon.com
- 3 Lipstick tubes – If using an old lipstick container one make sure it is clean, dried and sterilized.
- 3 drops peppermint essential oil

INSTRUCTIONS

- First, combine the mica, camelia seed oil, zinc oxide, and colorant to make your desired color while slowly incorporating the zinc oxide and rice flour to make the shade you prefer.
- Ensure there are no lumps and the powder is well dissolved with the oil.
- Melt the butter and waxes in a double boiler on low heat until melted.
- Add the colored oil mixture, mix well until melted.
- Pour in the empty lipstick tube as explained in the tutorial below.
- Put in the freezer for 15 minutes.
- Unmold slowly as per instructions on the previous page (see the how to make lipstick recipe for more details).
- Use within one year.

INDEX

AZUKI BEANS 123
ALMOND OIL 52, 69
ALOE VERA 29, 31, 39, 65, 123
APRICOT KERNEL OIL 71
ARROWROOT 36, 91
AVOCADO OIL 21, 53, 143
BEESWAX 35, 69, 71, 73, 75, 79, 81, 83, 91, 99, 101, 133, 135, 143, 145, 147
BEETROOT 145
CALENDULA 77
CAMELIA SEED OIL 61, 107, 109, 111, 155
CANDELILLA WAX 35, 137, 155
CASTOR OIL 133, 137, 145, 147, 149, 151
CARNAUBA WAX 35, 67, 137, 151, 155
CHAMOMILE ESSENTIAL OIL 31, 33, 6, 115
CHAMOMILE HYDROSOL 27, 105, 107
CLAY (BENTONITE, GREEN, PINK..) 95, 119, 125, 127, 129, 131
COCOA BUTTER 25, 53, 54, 65, 67, 71, 73, 77, 79, 83, 137, 147, 149
COCONUT OIL 22, 67, 79, 89, 133, 139, 145
COFFEE 79, 87, 125
CHARCOAL 127
GERANIUM ESSENTIAL OIL 33, 77, 79, 99, 105, 109, 127
GRAPESEED OIL 52, 65, 73, 113
HONEY 135, 147, 149
ORANGE BLOSSOM HYDROSOL 27, 101, 103, 111
JOJOBA OIL 21, 52, 83, 93, 103, 111, 113, 115, 127, 129, 143, 155
KUKUI OIL 22, 99
KOKUM BUTTER 25
LIQUID LECITHIN 37
LAVENDER ESSENTIAL OIL 33, 41, 59, 65, 71, 77, 91, 99, 103, 105, 113, 115, 127, 129

PINEAPPLE 85
PEPPERMINT ESSENTIAL OIL 33, 83, 89, 95, 133, 135, 143, 145, 147, 155
MANGO BUTTER 25, 54, 63, 79
MATCHA 121
RICE BRAN WAX 35, 155
ROSE HYDROSOL OR FLOWER WATER 99, 111, 131, 137
ROSEHIP OIL 22, 52, 111, 117, 127, 129
SALT 89
SACHA INCHI OIL 22, 105
SHEA BUTTER 25, 53, 54, 59, 61, 63, 67, 75, 77, 81, 83, 91, 93, 105, 107, 109, 145, 151, 155
SUNFLOWER OIL 21, 53, 67, 135, 145, 151, 155
SUGAR 87, 121
TEA TREE ESSENTIAL OIL 95, 127, 129
UCCUBA BUTTER 25, 109

Printed in Great Britain
by Amazon